The Secrets of Staying Young

Rosemary Conley CBE is the UK's most successful diet and fitness expert. Her diet and fitness books, videos and DVDs have consistently topped the bestseller lists with combined sales approaching nine million copies.

Rosemary has also presented more than 400 cookery programmes on television and has hosted several of her own TV series on BBC and ITV, including *Slim to Win with Rosemary Conley*, which was first broadcast in ITV Central and Thames Valley regions in 2007, with a new series in 2008. In 1999 Rosemary was made a Deputy Lieutenant of Leicestershire. In 2001 she was given the Freedom of the City of Leicester, and in 2004 she was awarded a CBE in the Queen's New Year Honours List for 'services to the fitness and diet industries'.

Together with her husband, Mike Rimmington, Rosemary runs five companies: Rosemary Conley Diet and Fitness Clubs, which operates an award-winning national network of almost 200 franchises running around 2000 classes weekly; Quorn House Publishing Ltd, which publishes Rosemary Conley *Diet & Fitness* magazine; Quorn House Media Ltd, which runs rosemaryconley.tv, an online TV channel; Rosemary Conley Licences Ltd; and Rosemary Conley Enterprises.

Rosemary has a daughter, Dawn, from her first marriage. Rosemary, Mike and Dawn are all committed Christians.

CENTURY

The Secrets of Staying Young

How to **feel** 30 years younger

Rosemary Conley

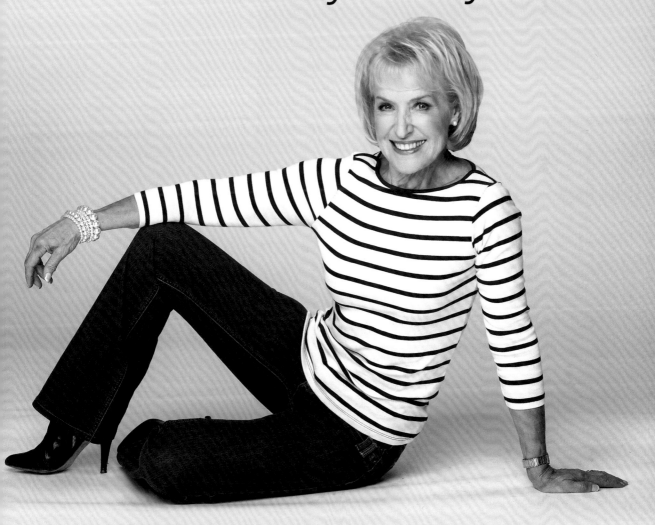

Published in the United Kingdom by Century in 2011

10 9 8 7 6 5 4 3 2 1

Century
Random House UK Limited
20 Vauxhall Bridge Road, London SW1V 2SA

Addresses for companies within The Random House Group Ltd can be found at
www.randomhouse.co.uk/offices.htm

The Random House UK Limited Reg. No. 954009

A CIP catalogue record for this book is available from the British Library

ISBN 9781846057311 (hb)
ISBN 9781846057328 (tpb)

Credits
Cover photographs by Alan Olley
Exercise photographs by Alan Olley
Photographs of Rosemary Conley, Mary Morris and Maureen Hyndman by Alan Olley
Food and product photographs by Clive Doyle
'After' photographs of slimmers Christine Cox, Jacki Franklin, Ginny Jones and Pat Wolfendon by Alan Olley
'After' photograph of slimmer Sylvia Willis by Martin Black
Edited by Jan Bowmer
Designed by Roger Walker

The Random House Group Limited supports The Forest Stewardship Council (FSC), the leading
international forest certification organisation. All our titles that are printed on Greenpeace
approved FSC certified paper carry the FSC logo. Our paper procurement policy can be found
at www.rbooks.co.uk/environment

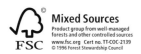

Mixed Sources
Product group from well-managed
forests and other controlled sources
www.fsc.org Cert no. TT-COC-2139
© 1996 Forest Stewardship Council
FSC

Printed and bound in Germany by Firmengruppe APPL, Aprinta Druck, Wemding

Contents

Acknowledgements

It has been a real pleasure to write this book because it's quite different from my usual diet books or cookbooks. It has made me think about what I have learned over the years from a lot of lovely people who have been an inspiration to me. I hope this book will encourage you to find the determination to put some of these things into practice so that you can feel younger for longer.

I want to say a big thank you to Dr Hilary Jones for his encouragement and help in putting together the health advice in this book and also to Professor Raj Persaud for his wisdom and insight into the psychological aspect of ageing and how to live younger for longer. These are two exceptional guys who never cease to inspire, educate and support me and I'm extremely grateful to them both.

Fitness expert Mary Morris and I have worked together for almost 18 years. Mary has been my fitness mentor and inspiration for as long as I can remember and I have learned so much from working alongside her. I don't think I have ever met anyone who has such a passion for helping others to become fitter and healthier by teaching people how to exercise safely and effectively. This book offers a variety of fitness advice and Mary helped me to put together the workouts for the different body shapes as well as the Forever Young Workout, which is designed to help us stay mobile as we reach the winter of our lives. Thank you, Mary, for everything you do and for everything you are.

Thank you to my wonderful chef, Dean Simpole-Clarke, who works so hard to create recipes for my magazine and my cookbooks, and who worked with me to create the recipes for this book.

Makeup artist extraordinaire Jane Tyler has transformed my face and my hair on many occasions over the years. We first met when I was appearing on ITV1's *This Morning* in the early 90s and since then we have worked together on endless fitness DVDs, magazine shoots and my own personal photo sessions. I've learned so much from Jane and she has taught me that knowing how to apply makeup and which brushes to use really can transform our looks. Thank you, Janie. You are a star!

Special thanks must go to my favourite personal photographer, Alan Olley. Alan seems to be able to capture me at my best and I am so grateful for that! We have worked together for years and always enjoy the photo shoots of successful slimmers for my *Diet & Fitness* magazine. Thank you, Alan, for always going the extra mile to get that special shot.

Thank you also to Clive Doyle for the still-life photography. Photographing food and products is a very different skill and you do it brilliantly, Clive.

Thanks are due to June Kenton, founder of Rigby and Peller, for her guidance on finding underwear to enhance the different body shapes; to franchisee Maureen Hyndman for so bravely volunteering to be the model for the hourglass shape workout and fashion shots; and to the successful slimmers who kindly gave their permission for their before and after photographs to be included. Well done to all of you for keeping your weight off after reaching your weight-loss goals. Thank you also to Siân Lee for sourcing the various products I mention so they could be photographed.

A big thank you to my PA, Diana Buchanan, for so carefully managing my manuscript as I was churning it out, and to our Executive Secretary Anja Zeman for her wizardry in calculating the calories in the diet plans. You are both brilliant.

Huge thanks must go to my long-suffering editor, Jan Bowmer, for her meticulous eye for detail and special talent for making everything in my books flow logically; to designer Roger Walker for his care and attention in making this book easy to follow for anyone who reads it. Thank you also to Susan Sandon and Gillian Holmes at the Random House Group for commissioning this book and making it possible for it to be published. Last but by no means least, I must thank my mother-in-law Jeanne. Now in her 90th year, Jeanne gamely agreed to be photographed doing the Forever Young Workout with me, much to the delight and amazement of everyone who was there. Jeanne, I want to be like you in 25 years' time! You really are an inspiration and a delight.

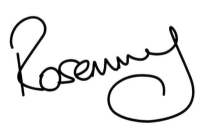

1
Being youthful
is fun

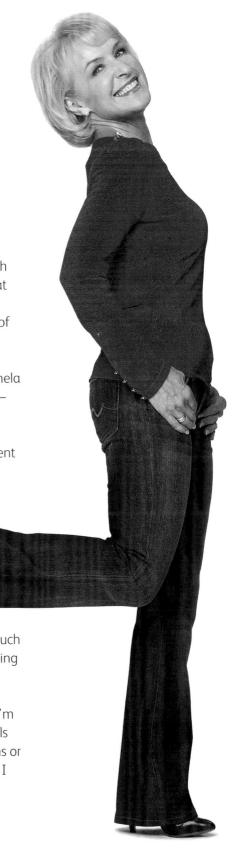

There's never been a better time to enjoy being fit and glamorous as a mature woman than right now. Thanks to mature female role models and reality television shows such as *Strictly Come Dancing*, it's universally acknowledged that age needn't be a barrier to looking good, nor an excuse. When actress Pamela Stephenson reached the semi-finals of *Strictly* in 2010 on her 61st birthday, the nation was full of admiration – not just for her energy, but also for her glamorous appearance and zest for life. At no time did Pamela make any excuses for her age, she just got on with the job – and did it magnificently. And that's what this book is all about: embracing our advancing years, maximising the opportunities to present ourselves as attractive and confident women, staying youthful and feeling fit in our maturity.

I'm not a fan of cosmetic surgery, nor am I a fitness fanatic. I'm not going to ask you to eat seaweed or even put tea bags on your eyelids – because I don't do that myself. I firmly believe that we can enhance our figure, minimise our wrinkles and create a good look by adopting some simple and healthy habits – such as eating well and getting our weight to a healthy level, being physically active and keeping our minds sharp by staying motivated and stimulated.

At the time of writing, my birth certificate states that I'm going to be 65 next birthday (Dec 2011), but my body feels like 35. I have bags of energy, I don't have aches and pains or mobility problems, I wear high heels most of the time and I love dressing up. In fact there's nothing I don't do now that I used to do 30 years ago. I love life and want to live to be 100!

Now, I'm not holding myself up as some great example of staying young – I have wrinkles, just like anyone else of my age, and that's not what this book is about. Rather it's about keeping our figures despite our advancing years, maintaining our facial muscle tone so we don't have a saggy face, and dressing to flatter our figures by camouflaging the worst bits and maximising the best features. I want to help you achieve a fit and healthy body as you progress into the autumn of your life and it's a goal that is very achievable.

Over the last 40 years I've had the privilege of working alongside some amazing experts in the field of nutrition, fitness, physical and mental health, as well as in cosmetics and fashion. I've learned so much from them and it has been a very exciting education. I've put that expertise into practice in my business, my *Diet & Fitness* magazine and in my personal life, so I know it works. Now I want you to have the benefit of that experience. I'm going to share with you the secrets of staying youthful and feeling 30 years younger. My aim is to give you as much information, help and encouragement as possible to enable you to live your life to the full – and to look and feel your youthful best.

Throughout this book I refer to a number of products that I've produced and developed over the years to help people to lose weight, become fitter, look younger and live more healthily. I work really hard to ensure that every product that enters my range is of high quality and that it works, and nothing is included unless I have personally tested it. You can be confident that I don't sell any product that is ineffective or that doesn't provide genuine value to the consumer. You can find full details of these products on my website (www.rosemaryconley.com). Also, I'll mention other products that I use and can recommend. These endorsements are given without inducement or reward and reflect my genuine opinion and experience.

2
What's happening to my body?

Once we understand what happens to the human body as we get older we can take action to counteract it. Our skin becomes looser and drier, our muscles smaller and weaker and our metabolic rate slower, making it easier for us to gain weight. Our eyesight becomes less sharp (though the bonus is that we can't see our wrinkles as easily!) and our memory fails us in a variety of ways. All of these things do happen and we can't avoid them completely but we can counter the effects of this bodily deterioration very effectively if we put our minds to making some lifestyle changes and adopting healthy habits that will keep us youthful.

If you are overweight, then I will help you lose your excess pounds and, I promise, you will feel years younger very quickly. After all, you could be walking around right now carrying the equivalent of your holiday suitcase, in which case there's no wonder you get tired, your joints hurt and you can't wait to kick off your shoes at the end of the day.

When I was preparing to write this book I decided to find out how it would

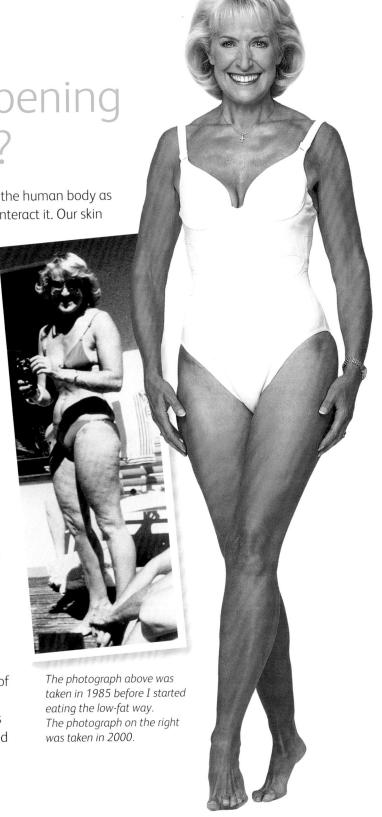

The photograph above was taken in 1985 before I started eating the low-fat way. The photograph on the right was taken in 2000.

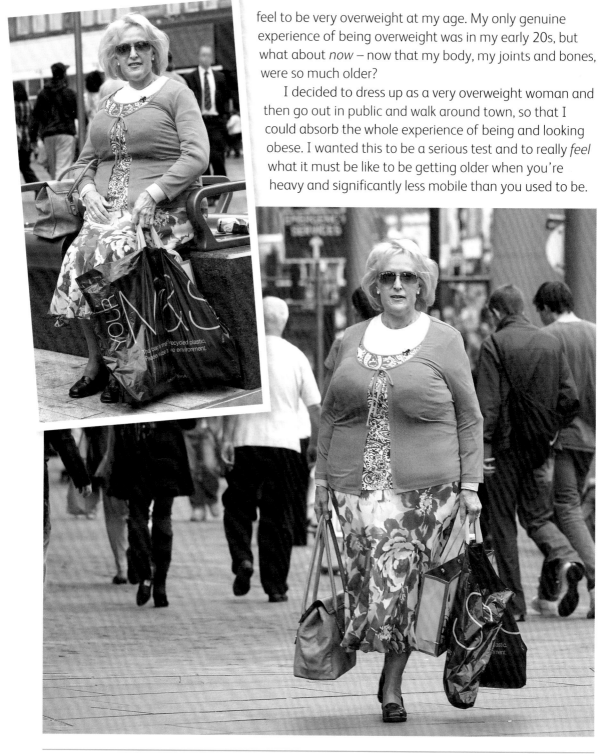

feel to be very overweight at my age. My only genuine experience of being overweight was in my early 20s, but what about *now* – now that my body, my joints and bones, were so much older?

I decided to dress up as a very overweight woman and then go out in public and walk around town, so that I could absorb the whole experience of being and looking obese. I wanted this to be a serious test and to really *feel* what it must be like to be getting older when you're heavy and significantly less mobile than you used to be.

To make my face fatter I had a prosthesis made, which gave me a couple of extra chins. I wore a 'fat jacket', which added considerable weight and bulk around my abdominal area, and had a 'Little Britain' fat suit cut down to fit my small 5ft 2in frame. By the time I was all 'assembled' I guess I must have looked about 4 stone overweight. In reality, the weight of all my additional bits and pieces of my costume added about 2½ to 3 stone. Instead of wearing my usual size-8 clothes, I wore a size-18 skirt and a size-16 top. To finish off the look, I bought some comfy flat shoes. I looked matronly and I felt awful – huge and unattractive, and embarrassed at stepping out in public.

I got out of the car and to my utter amazement no one batted an eyelid! As I made my way down from the car park to The Shires Shopping Centre in the middle of Leicester, other people who looked just like me got into the lift. It was strangely reassuring. Out on the street an elderly lady in a motorised scooter whizzed past me and looked even bigger than me. Nobody looked at her either.

I walked around the Clock Tower in the city centre and looked at the clothes in the shop windows, imagining what it would feel like to go in and ask to try something on. It must be so stressful to try to find something that fits a very oversized body. I felt so 'big' and took up so much room everywhere. Getting back into the car was really hard work. Walking had made my knees and feet ache and all I'd wanted to do all day was to sit down. Then when I eventually sat down, I found myself sitting with my feet apart to accommodate my vast stomach and realised why older women sat like that.

Going to the loo was a nightmare. I couldn't pull my tights up! There was so little room in the cubicle. How on earth do very overweight folk manage on an aircraft where the toilets are tiny? When I dropped something, picking it up again was a major operation. I could hardly breathe. Being so big was just awful and I felt 20 years older.

These were the physical inconveniences and emotions I felt, but what about the physiological damage it would have caused if my padding had been for real? If I truly were 4 stone overweight my blood pressure would be up, putting me at risk of having a heart attack or stroke; I would almost certainly have Type 2 diabetes, which can be life-threatening; my knees and hips would probably need replacing at some point and my back, feet and ankles would be killing me. Everyday activities would be hard to cope with. Even having a bath would be difficult, and the pace at which I did everything would seem so slow.

By the end of the day, I felt exhausted. I wouldn't have believed that I could exercise – after all, going upstairs was really difficult. I imagine it would all seem so hopeless and I'd probably write it off as 'I'm getting older and I just can't do what I used to. Get used to it.'

But it *so* doesn't need to be like that and this book will help you transform your life so that you live younger for longer.

We filmed my day in the fat suit from beginning to end and you can view it by logging on to www.rosemaryconley.tv/rosemary/fatsuit.

Use it or lose it

If you don't exercise at the moment, I'm going to encourage you to start, even if you do only a little bit of activity at the beginning. Getting fitter by doing some activity that you enjoy on a regular basis is the most effective youth-giving medicine you could ever have. It exercises the most important muscle in your body – your heart – and just like any other muscle, for instance the bicep muscle in your arm, if you exercise it regularly it will become bigger and stronger. The heart is the 'engine room' of the body, so getting it fit and strong provides the foundation for a fit and youthful future. Exercise also burns calories, which helps you to control your weight as well as dramatically improve your body shape.

There's a natural tendency for our bodies to 'head south' as we get older if we leave them to their natural path. Our boobs droop, our tummies get bigger, our waists thicken and our bottoms sag. It's not an attractive prospect for any of us, but we can reverse all these with a bit of effort. Better still, we can prevent it happening in the first place if we develop a healthy and active lifestyle from our 40s or 50s.

In our younger years we are more physically active because we *have* to be – carrying a child on one hip while reassembling a pushchair, carrying the shopping, chasing after the children, doing our household jobs before and after we go to work. Life is extremely hectic and our muscles get a great workout without going anywhere near a gym. As we get older the pace of life changes and with it our energy expenditure (calories spent), which is why we often gain weight. We may not be eating very differently from the way we've always done and so we can't understand why we gain weight and our body shape changes. It all seems so unfair.

Once we pass childbearing age, the body's metabolism slows down dramatically. In fact it starts slowing down from the age of 30. But we can counter this in two ways. We can stay fit so that our muscles remain strong, which will help us to maintain our metabolic rate. Secondly, we can keep our weight at a healthy level so that we are able to move around easily without becoming exhausted, and exercise and activity will then become a pleasure rather than a chore.

When I'm out and about I see folk of my age carrying several stone of excess weight and struggling to even walk. It's heartbreaking, because if only they could shed some weight they'd be able to walk around with ease and their whole life-quality would be totally transformed as well as their inner health.

So, in order of importance, to get yourself feeling youthful again, your first step is to SLIM DOWN.

They did it – so can you!

For further inspiration, take a look at the successful slimmers on the following pages. All these ladies, whose ages now range from 53 to 74, found a new lease of life after losing their excess weight and getting fitter. Not only did they transform their figures, but also their health and their energy levels – and they all look and feel more youthful.

Jacki Franklin

Jacki Franklin, 57, lost almost 4 stone at her local Rosemary Conley class and turned her life around. Jacki, from Suffolk, says: 'Losing weight and getting fitter was the best move I ever made. I've ditched my "granny knickers" and now wear size-12 skinny jeans. I feel years younger, and losing so much weight and getting fit has helped my health enormously. Now I can really enjoy being a grandmother and live life to the full.'

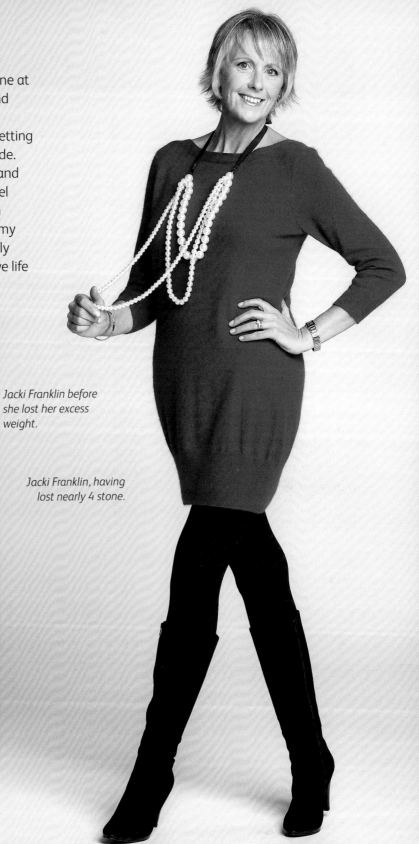

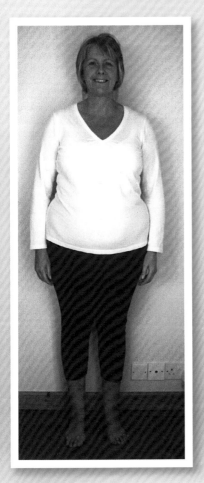

Jacki Franklin before she lost her excess weight.

Jacki Franklin, having lost nearly 4 stone.

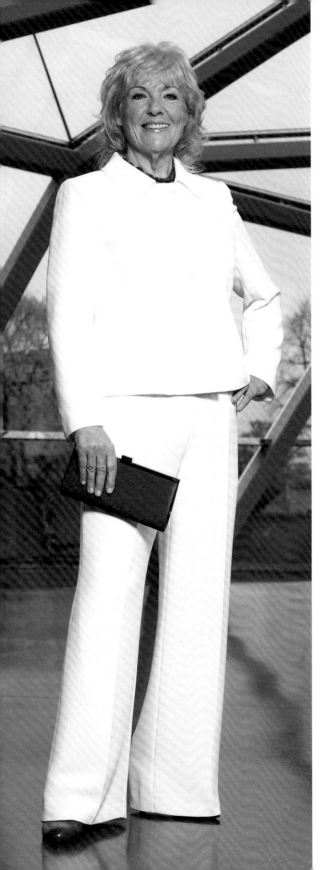

Ginny Jones

When Ginny Jones, 61, weighed over 21 stone she was virtually housebound. With an underactive thyroid, diabetes and almost crippled with arthritis, Ginny could barely shuffle a hundred yards with a walking stick. Her doctor warned her that her health was in serious jeopardy if she didn't lose weight. Ginny, from North Wales, joined her local Rosemary Conley class and in three years she lost 11st 4lb. She now fits into a size 12 instead of the size-34 clothes she used to wear and is always on the go. Ginny says: 'I can do so much more with my life now. I even go belly dancing once a week. Because I did so much exercise along with the diet, my skin is really well toned too. I really believe that doing this has saved my life.'

Right: *Ginny Jones when she weighed over 21 stone and wore size-34 clothes.*

Ginny Jones, having lost 11st 4lb.

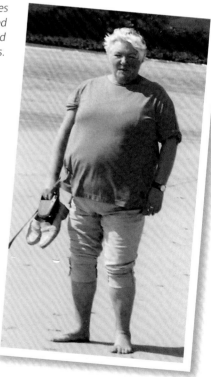

Sylvia Willis

Sylvia Willis is 74 and now feels younger than she did 40 years ago. Having shed 4st 8lb in 12 months at her local Rosemary Conley class, Sylvia, from Surrey, was so excited when she bought her first pair of jeans at the age of 69! Now, five years later and still slim, Sylvia says: 'I dance and live life to the full. I don't see why older people should act their age! I buy size-8 T-shirts from M&S and I now have a lovely size-10 swimming costume, which feels great. I hadn't felt comfortable in swimwear for years!'

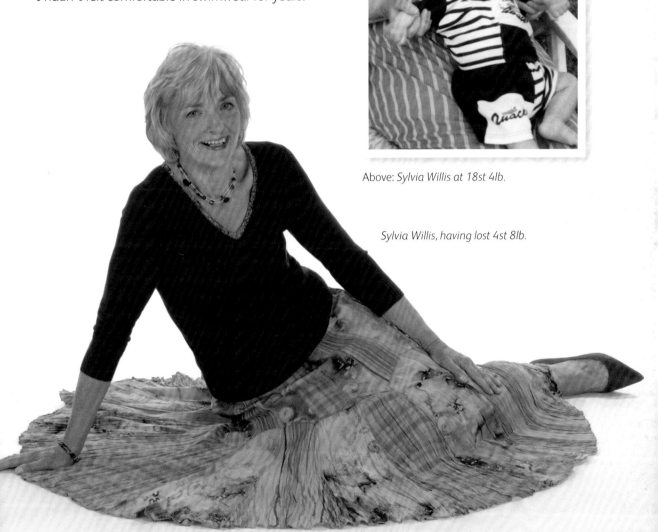

Above: *Sylvia Willis at 18st 4lb.*

Sylvia Willis, having lost 4st 8lb.

Christine Cox

Christine Cox, 54, had attempted to diet for years but suffered serious food cravings to the point she became obsessed with food. Vowing never to join another slimming club, she enrolled at a salsa class, not realising it was one of our Slim & Salsa classes! Christine, from Hertfordshire, went on to lose a couple of stone in a few months. She says: 'I'm in better shape now both physically and mentally than I've ever been. I'm not obsessed with food any more and for the first time in my life I'm happy with my body. I feel younger and physically free and my marriage has been rejuvenated.'

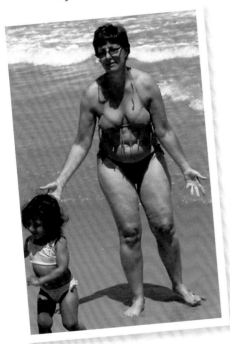

Above: *Christine Cox at 11 stone when she was obsessed with food.*

Christine Cox, having lost 2 stone.

Pat Wolfendon

Ward sister Pat Wolfendon, 53, from Lancashire, used to weigh 17st 9½lb. After years of chronic ill health and failed attempts at dieting, Pat joined her local Rosemary Conley class, where she lost an amazing 7st 4lb in just one year. Now Pat's a trim 10st 5lb and as her weight plummeted her confidence soared. She says: 'Before I lost weight I looked and felt like a fat blob. I had no self-respect and zero confidence. Now I can walk along the street full of confidence. I never stop smiling because life is so good!'

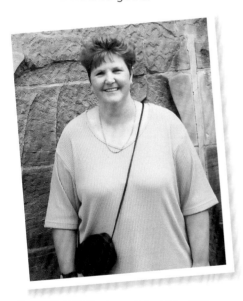

Above: *Pat Wolfendon weighed 17st 9½lb at her heaviest.*

Pat Wolfendon, having lost 7st 4lb.

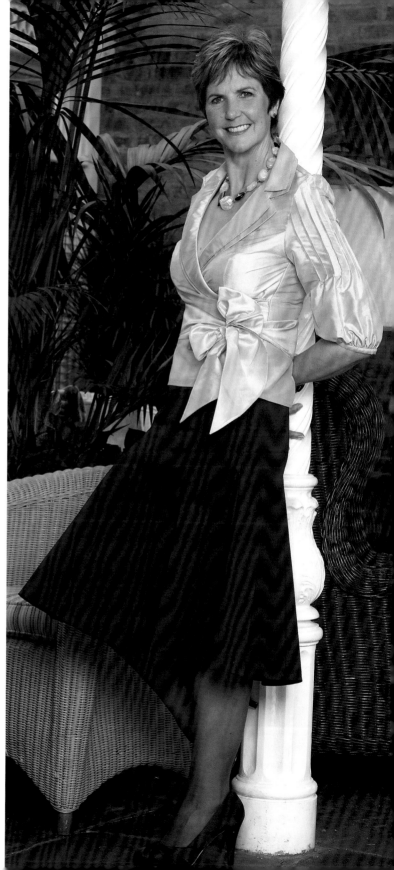

3
How to lose weight

If you are overweight, it's as if you have 'banked' too much food in your body's 'savings account' and you are storing those savings in the form of fat. To reverse that, you need to go on a spending spree of energy and deposit less food on a daily basis so you use up some of these savings. In other words, to lose weight you need to *eat less* and *do more*.

Losing weight is a simple matter of physics. *Eat* more calories than you spend, and you'll gain weight. *Spend* more calories than you eat, and you'll lose weight. It's as simple as that.

So what are calories? A kilocalorie is a unit of energy used by scientists to measure the energy value of the foods we eat and the energy we spend through activity. If you look at the nutrition panel printed on food packaging, the 'energy' value is given in kj (kilojoules) and kcal (kilocalories). The kcal (kilocalories) figure will tell you the number of calories per 100 grams of that product. For ease of reference, I'll simply refer to kilocalories as 'calories' or 'kcal'.

Every day your body spends calories just to stay alive. It's like a car with the engine constantly running and using fuel. Your heart beats continually until the day you die, your lungs expand and contract, your organs function continuously, your hair grows, your skin renews itself, and so on. Even if you stayed in bed all day and didn't move your body, you'd still burn calories just by staying alive. The number of calories you'd burn in this situation is your basal metabolic rate (BMR). For a woman aged over 60 and weighing about 10st 7lb, this figure will be about

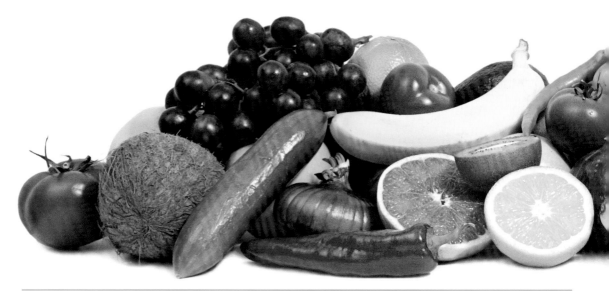

1200. The BMR of a man of the same weight and age will be slightly higher, at around 1350. If you weigh less than this, your BMR will be lower and, if you weigh more, it will be higher.

All my diets work on the principle of eating the number of calories that meets your basal metabolic needs. So if you have a BMR of 1200, I recommend you follow a diet of 1200 calories a day and combine it with extra activity. After four weeks on my Stay Young Diet, look up your personal BMR on the detailed charts on pages 218–219 and, from then on, base the daily calories in your weight-reducing plan on this figure. Once you reach your goal weight, the calories can be increased slightly to maintain your new weight.

By following a diet that has the same number of calories as your BMR you'll maximise your rate of weight loss, as you'll still be eating sufficient calories to meet your basic metabolic needs and yet eating considerably fewer calories than before to bring about a significant rate of weight loss. Add in some daily exercise and you'll speed up your weight loss as well as help your skin to shrink back very effectively and improve your overall health and fitness.

Eat low fat

Gram for gram, fat contains more than twice as many calories as carbohydrate or protein foods, and the fat you eat is very easily stored as fat on your body. If you eat a low-fat diet you can cut out loads of calories without eating less quantity of food. I recommend you only buy foods and products with 5 per cent or less fat content – something I've done for 25 years and I've never been so lean and healthy.

Cooking the low-fat way is easier than you might think and you can learn how to do it by logging on free to my web TV channel (www.rosemaryconley.tv) and watching chef Dean Simpole-Clarke demonstrate hundreds of low-fat recipes for you to enjoy. Just keep within your

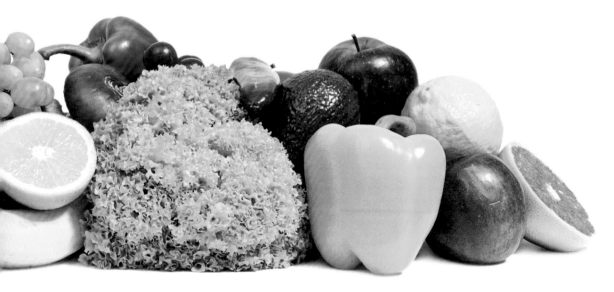

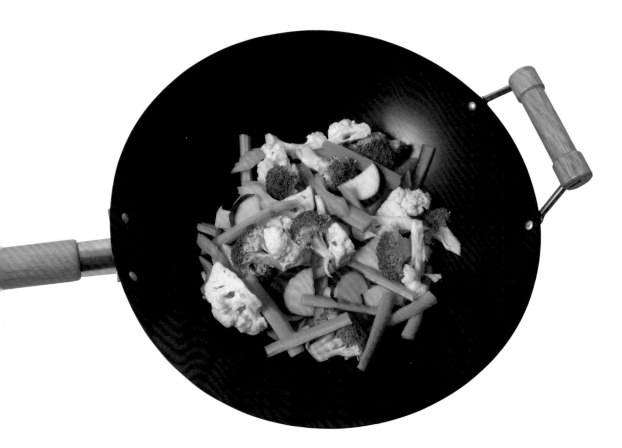

calorie allowance for each day and you will lose weight. Dean and I have written several low fat cookbooks together – check out my website for details.

You can cut out lots of fat calories just by making some simple adjustments to the way you prepare food. Instead of adding butter or margarine to your mashed potatoes, try substituting milk or low-fat plain yogurt. With a non-stick pan or wok, you can stir-fry any meat, fish, or vegetables without adding any fat or oil to the pan. It's important to remember that oil is 100 per cent fat and if you eat it you will end up wearing it!

When making sandwiches, spread your bread with low-fat dressings in preference to butter or margarine and save yourself lots of fat and calories. Branston pickle, low-fat mayonnaise, extra light soft cheese, HP sauce and horseradish sauce are great alternatives to butter or margarine and can be spread straight onto the bread.

The only foods exempt from my 5 per cent fat rule are oily fish like mackerel, herring and salmon; porridge oats and some lean cuts of meat, but by following the simple rule of thumb of eating low-fat foods you will transform your health and your figure. Eating a low-fat diet will also help lower your cholesterol levels and your blood pressure, help you sleep better, snore less, reduce heartburn dramatically and eliminate indigestion. You'll be amazed how soon you start to reap real benefits in the way you look and feel.

4
The Stay Young Diet

Your skin's health and the clarity of your eyes are greatly determined by what you eat and drink. Drink too much alcohol, and it will show in your face and eyes. Eat a poor diet and your skin will lack lustre and youthfulness. Eat well and your skin will glow with health, so your first step to looking good starts right here with what you put in your mouth.

The Stay Young Diet is based on foods that are rich in antioxidants in order to fight the free radicals waging war inside the body and which contribute to the ageing process. Fruit and vegetables that are high in antioxidants are easily recognised by their bright colour. These foods are also rich in life-giving vitamins and minerals. Oranges, tomatoes, peppers, blueberries, carrots and broccoli are positively bursting with anti-ageing antioxidants. Eat them regularly and you'll transform your health and your weight, and your skin will look more youthful and your eyes brighter.

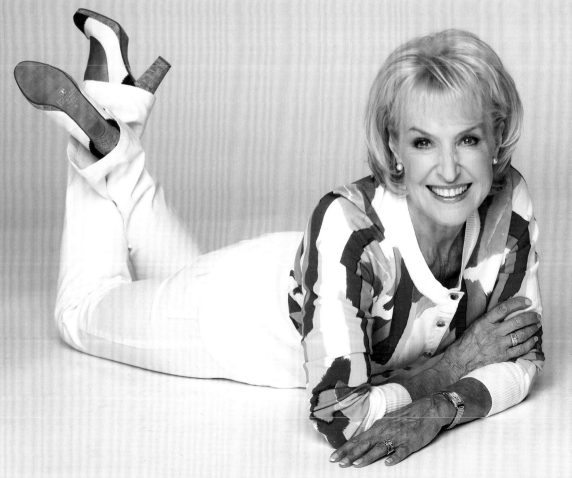

You can choose to follow the diet plan below and prepare your own meals, or turn to page 43 and follow my Stay Young Solo Slim® Diet, which is based on my healthy food range of ready meals, soups and snacks.

The Stay Young Diet

Daily Allowance

Weeks 1 and 2 (Stay Young Kick-Start Diet)

Breakfast	200 kcal
Mid-morning Power Snack	50 kcal
Lunch	300 kcal
Mid-afternoon Power Snack	50 kcal
Dinner	400 kcal
Milk allowance (450ml / ¾ pint skimmed or semi-skimmed milk)	200 kcal
TOTAL Weeks 1 and 2	**1200 kcal**

Weeks 3 and 4 add-ons

Alcoholic drink, dessert or snack	200 kcal (total)
TOTAL Weeks 3 and 4	**1400 kcal**

Diet notes
★ Water, low-cal drinks and tea and coffee (using milk from allowance) are unrestricted.
★ If you wish, you can eat your main meal at lunchtime.
★ All meals are interchangeable within each category.
★ The Power Snacks can be eaten mid-morning and mid-afternoon, as suggested, or at any time you choose.
★ Spare calories (from unused Power Snacks) can be saved up and used for a social occasion.
★ Aim to eat 5 portions of fruit and/or vegetables per day.
★ ☑ means suitable for vegetarians or vegetarian option is available.

Step 1: Weeks 1 and 2

Follow the 1200-calorie Stay Young Kick-Start eating plan for two weeks. Each day, select and eat a breakfast, lunch and dinner from the menus listed, plus two Power Snacks that can be eaten mid-morning and mid-afternoon or at any other time you choose. In addition, you should consume 450ml (¾ pint) skimmed or semi-skimmed milk each day, which can be taken with breakfast cereals and in tea and coffee throughout the day.

Make sure you do some form of exercise for around 20–30 minutes each day. Exercise such as walking, swimming, aerobics, dancing or playing sport is fine, but you should build into this two aerobics classes a week or follow one of my fitness DVDs twice a week. In Chapters 17 to 19 you will find a suggested weekly exercise plan to suit your body shape.

An aerobics class or an aerobic workout from one of my DVDs will work many of the muscles all over your body to ensure you gain good muscle strength and definition, which will help you achieve a youthful figure. Although walking and cycling are great fat-burners and are terrific for strengthening your legs, they will not use the muscles in your middle or upper body. An aerobics class, on the other hand, will give you a brilliant all-over workout. I teach just two classes a week and this has helped me to achieve and maintain a reasonably proportioned figure.

Exercise speeds up your metabolism for several hours beyond your workout, causing you to burn extra calories so that you lose weight faster, and it helps your skin to shrink and tone up as you slim down. So, if you want to see and feel results fast, stick to the diet and do the recommended activity.

Step 2: Weeks 3 and 4

After two weeks on the Stay Young Kick-Start Diet you can increase your daily allowance by 200 calories, to make a total of 1400 calories per day. You can take these extra calories in the form of alcohol or extras such as a dessert or a bedtime snack. Just ensure that the total doesn't exceed 200 calories. Alternatively, you can save up the extra calories over a week for a special occasion.

To enjoy maximum benefit to your rate of weight loss and your health, be sure to continue with the recommended 20–30 minutes of physical activity each day, including two aerobics sessions. Very soon you'll notice a real difference – not only in your fitness level, but also in the number of inches you lose from around your body. Remember to measure yourself every week to see the improvements in your figure.

Step 3: Week 5 onwards

After four weeks on the Stay Young Diet you'll be significantly slimmer and will feel much fitter as a result of the exercise.

Depending on your weight, age and gender, you may now increase your daily calorie allowance, depending on your BMR. Consult the charts on pages 218–219 to recalculate the daily calorie allowance that is appropriate to you personally, and continue on this daily intake until you lose about another 7lb, at which point your calorie allowance will need to be adjusted again to take account of the weight you have lost. Continue with your daily physical activity and make it part of your everyday lifestyle. Do this and you will stay younger for longer.

The Stay Young Kick-Start Diet

Daily Allowance: 1200 calories

Breakfast	200 kcal
Mid-morning Power Snack	50 kcal
Lunch	300 kcal
Mid-afternoon Power Snack	50 kcal
Dinner	400 kcal
Milk allowance (450ml / ¾ pint skimmed or semi-skimmed milk)	200 kcal
Unlimited water, low-cal drinks, tea and coffee (with milk from allowance)	

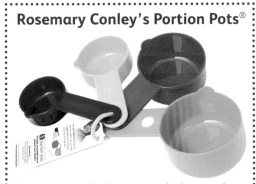

Rosemary Conley's Portion Pots®

Portion control is key to weight loss, and these innovative pots make measuring everyday food simple! Each set comes with an informative guide.

Order from www.rosemaryconley.com

DAY 1

Breakfast ☑
- 1 yellow Portion Pot® (125ml) fresh orange juice
- 1 small can tomatoes, boiled well to reduce, served on 2 medium slices toasted wholegrain bread

Mid-morning Power Snack ☑
- 90g fresh blueberries

Lunch ☑
- 1 pouch **Solo Slim® Carrot and Coriander Soup** plus 1 small wholegrain roll
- Fresh fruit salad – e.g. blueberries, grapes, pineapple, papaya, mango (175g total)

Mid-afternoon Power Snack ☑
- 1 brown Ryvita spread with extra light soft cheese (e.g. Philadelphia Extra Light) plus 2 cherry tomatoes

Dinner
- **Chicken and Chilli Stir-Fry** (see recipe)
- Served with 40g (dry weight) basmati rice, boiled

Chicken and Chilli Stir-Fry

SERVES 1 *(for more than 1 serving, just multiply the ingredients)*
Per serving: 247 calories 2.4g fat (0.4% fat) excluding rice
403 calories 3.4g fat (0.6% fat) including rice

1 skinless chicken breast (approx. 110g), chopped
1 garlic clove, crushed
½ red onion, coarsely chopped
2 celery sticks, chopped
½ fresh chilli, deseeded and finely chopped
½ each green, red and yellow peppers,
    cut into bite-sized squares
6 button mushrooms, halved
2cm piece fresh root ginger,
    peeled and finely grated
½ bunch fresh coriander, coarsely
    chopped
Freshly ground black pepper,
    to taste

For the sauce
1 tbsp chilli and ginger
    dipping sauce
1 tbsp soy sauce

For serving
40g (dry weight) basmati
    rice
1 vegetable stock cube

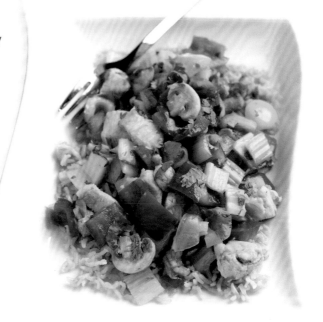

1 Preheat a non-stick wok. When hot, add the chopped chicken breast, the crushed garlic and freshly ground black pepper. Toss the chicken to seal it on all sides and cook for 12 minutes.
2 Meanwhile, put the rice on to cook in a pan of boiling water with the vegetable stock cube added.
3 When the chicken is almost cooked, add the chopped red onion and the celery and heat through. Then add the chopped chilli, chopped peppers and mushrooms and toss well to heat through. When all the ingredients are hot, add the grated ginger and then stir in the chilli and ginger dipping sauce and soy sauce.
4 Drain the rice. Just before serving the chicken, stir in the fresh coriander, coarsely chopped with scissors. Serve with the boiled basmati rice and additional soy sauce if desired.

Note: It's important not to overcook the fresh vegetables in this stir-fry, so start to boil the rice while the chicken is cooking and only add the vegetables to the chicken 3 minutes before serving.

DAY 2

Breakfast ☑
■ Energy Muesli (prepare the night before): Take 15g porridge oats, 10g sultanas, 4 chopped almonds, 1 apple, coarsely grated, 1 carrot, coarsely grated, and mix with 50g low-fat natural yogurt

Mid-morning Power Snack ☑
■ ½ Rosemary Conley Low Gi Nutrition Bar, any flavour, or 1 piece fresh fruit

Lunch
■ **Tropical Prawn Salad** (see recipe)

Mid-afternoon Power Snack ☑
■ ½ Rosemary Conley Low Gi Nutrition Bar, any flavour, or 1 piece fresh fruit

Dinner
■ 1 pouch **Solo Slim® Tomato Soup** or similar (max. 168 kcal per serving)
■ 80g roast chicken served with 80g carrots, 80g broccoli, 2 (50g total) dry-roasted sweet potatoes and a little gravy made with gravy powder

For details of how to order Rosemary Conley's Solo Slim® ready meals and soups, see page 48.

Tropical Prawn Salad

SERVES 2
Per serving: 285 calories 2.4g fat (0.4% fat)

For the sauce
2 tbsps extra light mayonnaise
1 tbsp tomato ketchup
2cm piece fresh root ginger, peeled
  and finely grated

For the salad
Selection of rocket and lamb's
  lettuce leaves
200g large cooked shelled prawns
¼ fresh pineapple, peeled and cut
  into squares
½ small papaya, peeled, deseeded and cut
  into chunks
½ mango, peeled and sliced away from
  the stone, then cut into chunks
10 cherry tomatoes, halved
2cm piece cucumber, peeled and chopped
½ red onion, finely chopped
¼ each red, green, yellow peppers,
  chopped
2 celery sticks, chopped

1   Make up the sauce by mixing the extra
    light mayonnaise with the tomato
    ketchup and root ginger.
2   Place a few salad leaves in 2 serving
    dishes. Layer some of the prawns and
    the other ingredients on top and drizzle
    with some of the sauce. Add more
    leaves and a further layer of ingredients,
    and continue layering until they are
    used up. Drizzle the remaining sauce
    over the top.

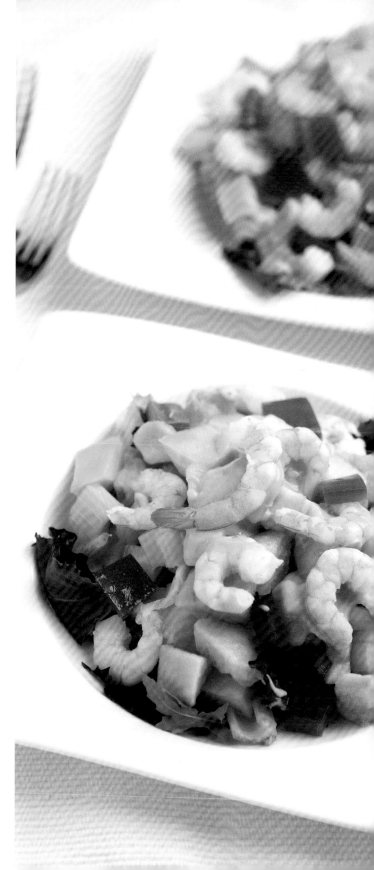

DAY 3

Breakfast ☑
- 200g Total 2% fat Greek yogurt served with 100g fresh blueberries

Mid-morning Power Snack ☑
- 1 brown Ryvita spread with extra light soft cheese plus 2 cherry tomatoes

Lunch ☑
- **Spicy Butternut Squash Soup** (see recipe) or ready-made alternative (max. 77 kcal per serving)
- Plus 1 small wholegrain roll

Spicy Butternut Squash Soup

SERVES 4
Per serving: 77 calories 1g fat (0.5% fat)

1 small butternut squash
115g fresh young carrots, washed and sliced
2 medium onions, chopped
2 garlic cloves, crushed
2 celery sticks, chopped
1–2 tsps medium curry powder (e.g. tandoori mix)
1.2 litres (2 pints) vegetable stock
2 bay leaves
Freshly ground black pepper, to taste

For serving
1 tbsp 0% fat Greek yogurt

1   Preheat a large non-stick saucepan.
2   Cut the squash in half lengthways. Remove the seeds with a spoon and discard. Using a sharp vegetable knife, peel away the thick skin and cut the flesh into chunks.
3   Place the squash and the other vegetables in the hot pan and dry-fry for 4–5 minutes, until they soften and start to colour.
4   Stir in the curry powder and cook for 1 minute, keeping the mixture moving to prevent it catching on the bottom of the pan. Gradually pour in the vegetable stock, stirring continuously, then add the bay leaves and bring to the boil.

5 Reduce the heat and simmer until the vegetables are tender.
6 Allow the soup to cool slightly, remove the bay leaves, then transfer the soup to a food processor or liquidiser and liquidise until smooth. Return the soup to the pan and adjust the consistency with a little extra stock. Season to taste with salt and black pepper and serve with a swirl of Greek yogurt on top.

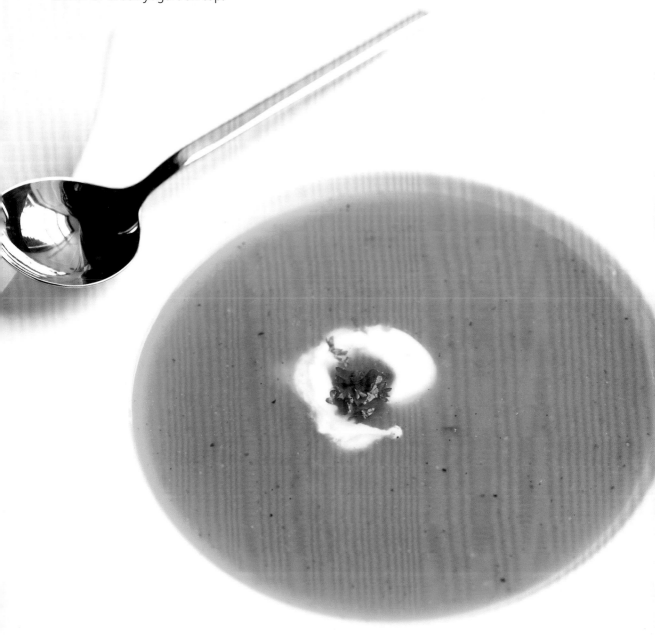

Mid-afternoon Power Snack ☑

2 satsumas

Dinner

■ 80g fresh salmon steak, grilled, microwaved or baked, served with 130g mangetout and 115g boiled new potatoes (with skins). Top with 1 tbsp extra light mayonnaise mixed with 1 tsp chilli and ginger dipping sauce

■ Eton Mess: 1 meringue basket, broken up, mixed with 1 tbsp 2% fat Greek yogurt and 10 fresh raspberries

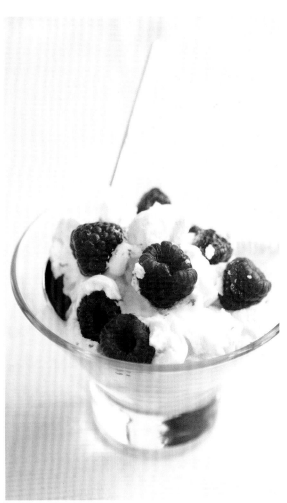
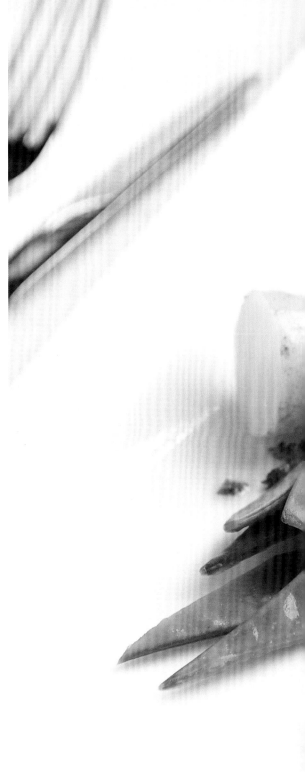

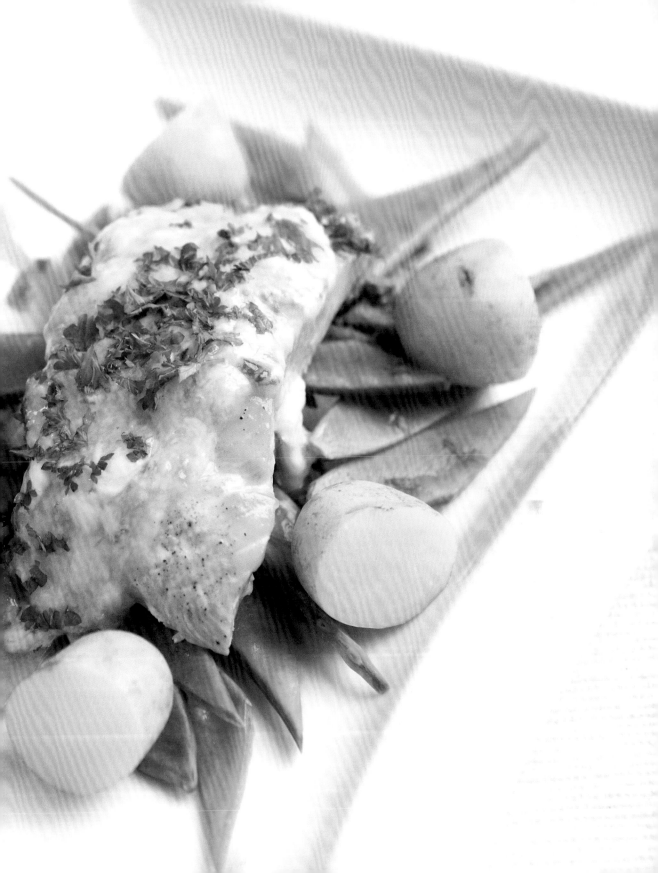

DAY 4

Breakfast ☑
- Soak 15g All-Bran overnight in 100g low-fat plain yogurt with 4 chopped almonds, 10 sultanas and 1 tsp honey. When ready to eat, add a little milk from allowance if the consistency is too thick

Mid-morning Power Snack ☑
- 2 satsumas

Lunch ☑
- 1 can any soup (max. 170 kcal and 5% fat) plus 1 medium slice wholegrain bread, toasted
OR
- 1 pouch **Solo Slim® Three Bean and Chorizo Soup** plus 1 medium slice wholegrain bread, toasted

Mid-afternoon Power Snack ☑
- 1 brown Ryvita spread with Marmite and topped with 3 sliced cherry tomatoes

Dinner
- **Thai Chicken** (see recipe)
- Served with 50g (dry weight) basmati rice per person and a mixed salad
OR
- 1 pouch **Solo Slim® Thai Chicken Curry** plus a small salad of mixed leaves, cherry tomatoes, chopped cucumber, red onion, chopped peppers and 3 baby beetroot tossed in very low-fat calorie dressing
- 1 medium banana

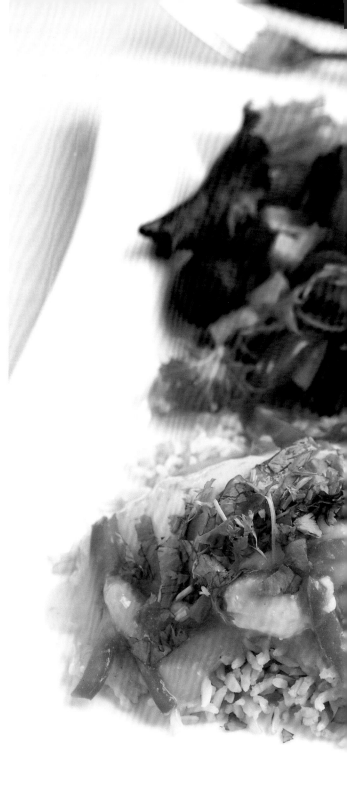

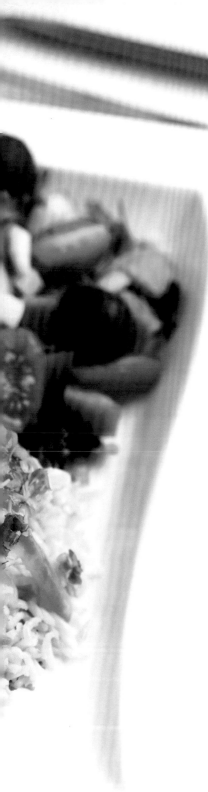

Thai Chicken

SERVES 4
Per serving: 203 calories 2.2g fat (0.6 % fat) excluding rice
408 calories 2.4g fat (0.6 % fat) including rice

4 × 100g skinned chicken breasts
1 red pepper, finely sliced
6 spring onions, finely chopped
6 plum tomatoes skinned, deseeded and diced
1 green chilli, deseeded and finely chopped
Zest and juice of 2 limes
2 garlic cloves, crushed
1 tsp ground cumin
1 tsp ground coriander
1 tbsp cornflour
300ml (½ pint) pineapple juice
Salt and freshly ground black pepper, to taste
Chopped fresh coriander, to garnish

For serving
220g (dry weight) basmati rice
1 vegetable stock cube
Mixed salad

1 Preheat the oven to 190°C, 375°F, Gas Mark 5.
2 Place the chicken in an ovenproof dish and season on both sides with salt and pepper.
3 Place the red pepper, spring onions and tomatoes in a bowl. Add the chilli, lime juice and zest, garlic, cumin and coriander and combine well.
4 Dissolve the cornflour in the pineapple juice and pour over the vegetables and spices. Mix well and season with salt and pepper. Pour the vegetables, with the juice, over the chicken and bake in the oven for 30–35 minutes.
5 While the chicken is in the oven, cook the rice in a pan of boiling water with the vegetable stock cube, then drain.
6 Transfer the chicken to serving plates. Garnish with fresh coriander and serve with the boiled rice and a side salad.

DAY 5

Breakfast ☑
- 1 yellow Portion Pot® (125ml) fresh orange juice
- 1 egg, boiled or poached, plus 1 slice wholegrain bread, toasted, spread with Marmite

Mid-morning Power Snack ☑
- ½ Rosemary Conley Low Gi Nutrition Bar, any flavour, or 1 piece fresh fruit

Lunch ☑
- 1 × 150g baked sweet potato topped with 140g baked beans or 70g grated Rosemary Conley's 5% fat Mature Cheese or 80g tuna mixed with extra light mayonnaise and 1 tbsp sweetcorn

Mid-afternoon Power Snack ☑
- ½ Rosemary Conley Low Gi Nutrition Bar, any flavour, or 1 piece fresh fruit

Dinner
- **Pork in Spicy Yogurt Sauce** (see recipe)
- Served with 55g (dry weight) basmati rice, boiled, and a salad

Pork in Spicy Yogurt Sauce

SERVES 4
Per serving: 190 calories 4.7g fat (2.3% fat) excluding rice
395 calories 5.1g fat (2% fat) including rice

4 × 100g lean pork steaks
8 tbsps low-fat natural yogurt
1 tbsp mild curry powder
2 tbsps mango chutney
1 red chilli, finely chopped
1 tbsp chopped fresh coriander
1 tbsp chopped fresh mint
Salt and freshly ground black pepper, to taste

For serving
220g (dry weight) basmati rice
1 vegetable stock cube
Salad

1 Preheat the grill to high.
2 Remove any visible fat from the pork steaks. Place the steaks in a shallow, heatproof dish.
3 Combine the remaining ingredients in a bowl to make the sauce. Spread both sides of the pork steaks with the sauce and place under a hot grill for 8–10 minutes each side.
4 While the steaks are under the grill, cook the rice in a pan of boiling water with the vegetable stock cube added, then drain.
5 Serve the steaks with the boiled rice and a salad.

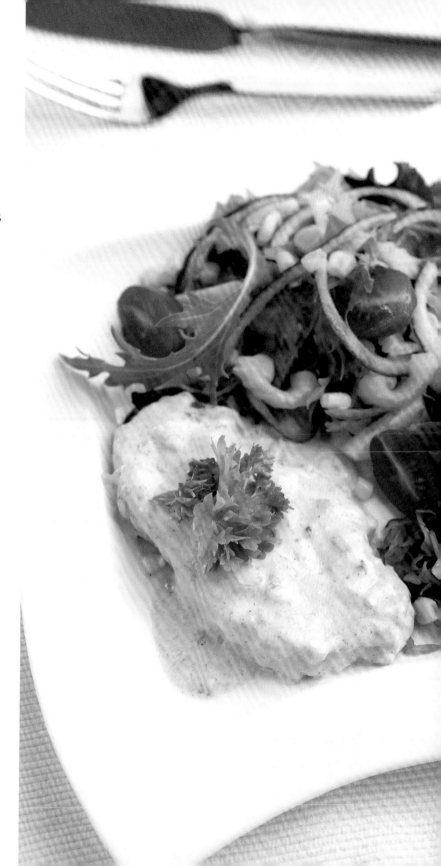

DAY 6

Breakfast ☑
- 1 yellow Portion Pot® (125ml) fresh orange juice
- 1 blue Portion Pot® (35g) porridge oats cooked in water and left overnight. Reheat and serve with milk from allowance and 1 tsp runny honey

Mid-morning Power Snack ☑
- 2 satsumas

Lunch
- 1 pouch **Solo Slim® Carrot and Coriander Soup** or similar (max. 78 kcal per serving)
- 3 brown Ryvita crispbreads spread with Philadelphia Extra Light soft cheese and topped with 25g smoked salmon or 50g wafer thin ham

Mid-afternoon Power Snack ☑
- 80g black seedless grapes

Dinner
- **Spaghetti Bolognese** (see recipe)

OR

- 1 pouch **Solo Slim® Pasta Bolognese** plus a small salad

Spaghetti Bolognese

SERVES 4
Per serving: 398 calories 8.9g fat (2% fat)

300g lean minced beef
2 garlic cloves, crushed
1 large onion, finely diced
2 medium carrots, coarsely grated
2 beef stock cubes
2 × 400g cans chopped tomatoes
2 tbsps tomato purée
1 tbsp chopped fresh mixed herbs (e.g. oregano, marjoram, basil, parsley)
225g (dry weight) spaghetti
1 vegetable stock cube
Freshly ground black pepper, to taste
Chopped fresh herbs, to garnish

1 Preheat a large, non-stick pan. Add the minced beef and dry-fry until it starts to change colour.
2 Remove the mince from the pan and wipe out the pan with kitchen paper. Return the meat to the pan, add the garlic and onion and continue cooking for a further 2–3 minutes, stirring well. Add the grated carrots and crumble the beef stock cubes over the top. Add the tomatoes, purée and mixed herbs, then mix well to allow the stock cubes to dissolve. Reduce the heat to a gentle simmer, season to taste, then cover with a lid and continue to cook for 30 minutes, until the sauce thickens.
3 Meanwhile, bring a large pan of water to the boil with the vegetable stock cube added. Add the spaghetti and cook for 12–15 minutes until the spaghetti is soft but slightly firm in the centre. Drain through a colander.
4 Arrange the spaghetti on warmed plates and pour the sauce on top. Garnish with fresh herbs.

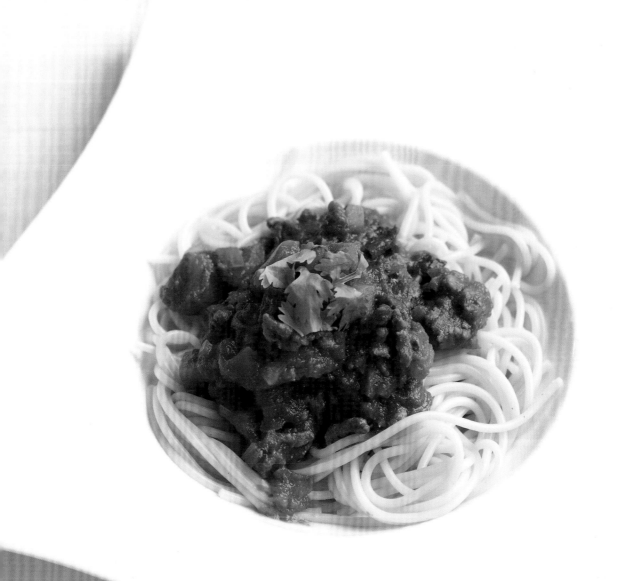

DAY 7

Breakfast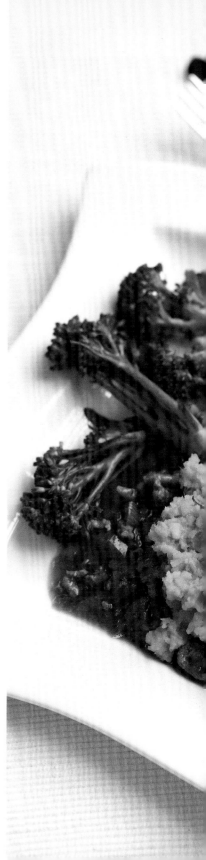
■ 1 green Portion Pot® (50g) Special K cereal served with milk from allowance and 1 tsp sugar

Mid-morningPower Snack
■ 2 satsumas

Lunch
■ Large salad of mixed dark green leaves – watercress, rocket, lamb's lettuce, etc. – topped with grated raw carrot, 10 cherry tomatoes, halved, 30g baby beetroot, sliced red, green and yellow peppers, sliced button mushrooms and 1 tbsp sweetcorn. Add 50g wafer thin ham, beef or chicken, low-fat cottage cheese or cold baked beans and serve with a little extra light mayonnaise

Mid-afternoon Power Snack
■ 1 Comice pear

Dinner
■ **Cottage Pie** (see recipe)
■ Served with 115g broccoli and 115g carrots

Cottage Pie

SERVES 2
Per serving: 400 calories 11.1g fat (2.8% fat)

2 large (300g total) sweet potatoes
1 vegetable stock cube
200g extra lean minced beef
1 onion, finely chopped
1 large carrot, grated
1 tbsp gravy powder
1 beef stock cube
A little milk from daily allowance
Freshly ground black pepper, to taste

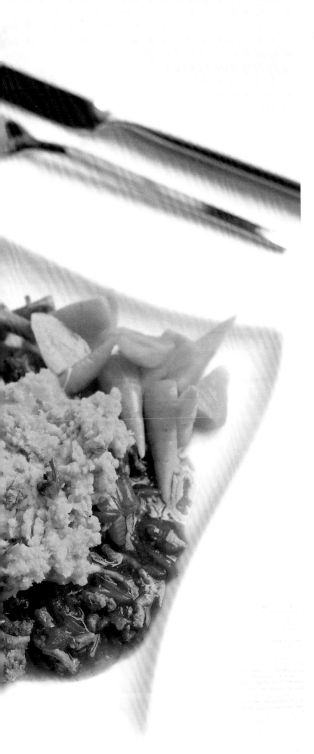

For serving
115g broccoli
115g carrots

1   Peel the potatoes, cut into small chunks and boil in water with the vegetable stock cube. When cooked, drain the potatoes, reserving the cooking water for the gravy later.

2   Meanwhile, preheat a non-stick wok or frying pan. Add the mince and dry-fry until it changes colour. Drain the mince through a colander, reserving the juices in a gravy separator. Return the mince to the pan and add the chopped onion and cook until soft. Add the grated carrot and mix well, then turn off the heat.

3   Preheat the oven to 200°C, 400°F, Gas Mark 6.

4   Start to make the gravy by mixing the gravy powder with a little cold water in a pan, then crumble in the beef stock cube. Pour in 300ml of the reserved potato cooking water and stir well. Slowly heat, stirring continuously to prevent the gravy from going lumpy. When boiling, add some gravy into the mince and vegetable pan, then pour the mince and vegetables into a pie dish.

5   Mash the potatoes, adding a little milk from your allowance and some freshly ground black pepper, until smooth and quite soft.

6   Carefully pile the mashed potato on top of the mince, making sure the mince is sealed to the edges to prevent the gravy bubbling out during cooking.

7   Place the cottage pie in the oven for 20 minutes. Serve with the broccoli and carrots and the remaining gravy.

Useful store cupboard staples

Breakfast cereals
All-Bran
Special K
Porridge oats

Canned foods
Baked beans
Chopped tomatoes

Condiments and flavourings
Black peppercorns
Marmite
Mustard
Pickle
Salt

Dressings
Hellmann's Extra Light Mayonnaise
Oil-free dressing
Very low fat dressing

Gravy powder
Bisto

Herbs and spices
Chilli powder
Dried oregano
Mixed dried herbs

Jams
Honey
Marmalade
Sugar-free jam

Pasta
Pasta shapes of choice
Spaghetti

Sauces
Fruity sauce
Tomato ketchup
Tomato purée
Soy sauce

Stock cubes
Beef
Chicken
Vegetable

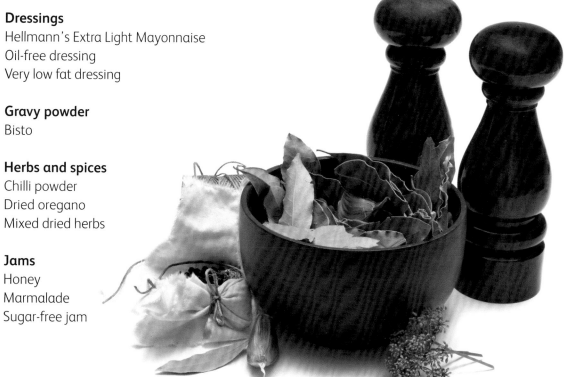

The Stay Young Solo Slim® Diet

Some people find it much easier to have their diet meals already prepared and calorie counted and, with this in mind, we created my Solo Slim® range of delicious, natural ready meals and soups. Last year I organised a trial of 30 volunteers who ate Solo Slim® for four weeks. They lost an average of 1st 1lb (15lb) in the 28 days. Here's a 7-day 1200-calorie diet plan designed around these meals, which have been selected because of their high antioxidant content. You can even order a Rosemary Conley Stay Young Solo Slim® Healthy Food Box (see pages 48–49), based on this selection. The Food Box also contains a pack of my low-fat Mature Cheese and the box is delivered direct to your door. All you have to do is provide your own breakfasts, the accompaniments to your ready meals – such as vegetables, potatoes and rice – and fresh fruit, following the suggestions given in the diet plan, plus your 450ml (¾ pint) daily milk allowance to complete your week's menu.

The diet is based on the same principles as the Stay Young Diet (1200 calories for the first two weeks and 1400 calories for weeks three and four. After week four, if you want to continue to lose weight, check your BMR on the charts on pages 218–9 to find your new personal calorie allowance and then adjust your daily calorie intake accordingly). It couldn't be easier and it's ideal for anyone who's dieting alone or who wants to eat different foods from the rest of the family.

The Stay Young Solo Slim® Diet

Daily Allowance

Weeks 1 and 2 (Stay Young Solo Slim® Kick-Start Diet)

Breakfast	200 kcal
Mid-morning Power Snack	50 kcal
Lunch	300 kcal
Mid-afternoon Power Snack	50 kcal
Dinner	400 kcal
Milk allowance (450ml/¾ pint skimmed or semi-skimmed milk)	200 kcal
TOTAL Weeks 1 and 2	**1200 kcal**

Weeks 3 and 4 add-ons

Alcoholic drink, dessert or snack	200 kcal (total)
TOTAL Weeks 3 and 4	**1400 kcal**

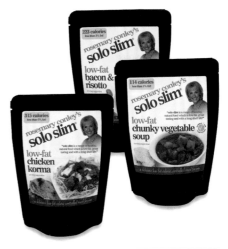

The Stay Young Solo Slim® Kick-Start Diet

This 7-day Stay Young Solo Slim® Kick-Start diet plan is based on 1200 calories per day. Don't forget to include your daily milk allowance of 450ml (¾ pint) skimmed or semi-skimmed milk.

DAY 1

Breakfast ☑
- 1 blue Portion Pot® (35g) porridge oats cooked in water served with 10 sultanas and milk from allowance

Mid-morning Power Snack ☑
- 2 satsumas

Lunch ☑
- 1 pouch **Solo Slim® Low-Fat Carrot and Coriander Soup** plus a small wholegrain bread roll
- 100g fresh fruit salad

Mid-afternoon Power Snack ☑
- 1 satsuma and 1 kiwi fruit

Dinner
- 1 pouch **Solo Slim® Low-Fat Chicken Hotpot** plus 100g broccoli and 100g cabbage or carrots
- 1 low-fat yogurt (max. 100 kcal and 5% fat)

Rosemary Conley's Solo Slim® ready meals and soups can be heated in the microwave or emptied into a saucepan or casserole dish and heated on the hob or in the oven.

Diet notes
- ★ Water, low-cal drinks and tea and coffee (using milk from allowance) are unrestricted.
- ★ If you wish, you can eat your main meal at lunchtime.
- ★ All meals are interchangeable within each category, so you can repeat your favourite ones if you like.
- ★ The Power Snacks can be eaten mid-morning and mid-afternoon, as suggested, or at any time you choose.
- ★ Spare calories (from unused Power Snacks) can be saved up and used for a social occasion.
- ★ Aim to eat 5 portions of fruit and/or vegetables per day.
- ★ ☑ means suitable for vegetarians or vegetarian option is available.

DAY 2

Breakfast ☑
- 2 Weetabix or Shredded Wheat served with milk from allowance plus 1 tsp sugar

Mid-morning Power Snack ☑
- 1 fresh pear or mini banana

Lunch ☑
- 1 pouch **Solo Slim® Low-Fat Minestrone Soup**
- 2 Ryvitas spread with 1 tsp very-low-fat mayonnaise and topped with 25g grated **Rosemary Conley's low-fat Mature Cheese** and 1 sliced tomato

Mid-afternoon Power Snack ☑
- 1 small apple or orange

Dinner
- 1 pouch **Solo Slim® Low-Fat Mushroom Soup**
- 1 pouch **Solo Slim® Low-Fat Chilli and Rice**

DAY 3

Breakfast ☑
- ½ fresh grapefruit plus 1 medium-sized egg, boiled or poached, served with 1 slice wholegrain bread, toasted and spread with Marmite

Mid-morning Power Snack ☑
- 280g slice honeydew melon (weighed with skin)

Lunch ☑
- 1 pouch **Solo Slim® Low-Fat Chunky Vegetable Soup**
- Large salad and 100g chicken/beef/ham or 40g **Rosemary Conley's low-fat Mature Cheese** plus 1 tsp very-low-fat mayonnaise

Mid-afternoon Power Snack ☑
- Chop 1 peeled carrot, 2 sticks celery and 1 × 5cm piece cucumber and serve with a dip made with 1 tsp very-low-fat mayonnaise and a pinch of chilli powder

Dinner ✓
- 1 pouch **Solo Slim® Low-Fat Carrot and Coriander Soup**
- 1 pouch **Solo Slim® Low-Fat Tomato and Vegetable Pasta** plus a small salad tossed in fat-free dressing
- 100g fresh fruit salad topped with 1 tsp Total 0% fat Greek yogurt

DAY 4

Breakfast ✓
- 1 × 100g pot low-fat natural yogurt (max. 75 kcal and 5% fat) mixed with 1 tbsp unsweetened muesli and 1 red Portion Pot® (115g) fresh raspberries

Mid-morning Power Snack ✓
- 280g slice honeydew melon (weighed with skin)

Lunch ✓
- 1 pouch **Solo Slim® Low-Fat Lentil Soup**
- 1 slice wholegrain bread spread with very-low-fat mayonnaise made into an open sandwich with 25g grated **Rosemary Conley's low-fat Mature Cheese**, 1 large sliced tomato, salad leaves, 1 sliced red onion and 4 slices cucumber

Mid-afternoon Power Snack ✓
- 75g seedless grapes

Dinner
- 1 pouch **Solo Slim® Low-Fat Tomato Soup**
- 1 pouch **Solo Slim® Low-Fat Beef Casserole** plus 100g broccoli or cabbage

Rosemary Conley's Solo Slim® ready meals and soups are made from 100 per cent fresh, natural ingredients with no E numbers or additives. They can be stored at room temperature with no need for refrigeration.

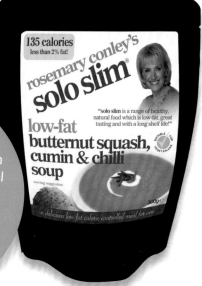

135 calories less than 2% fat!

rosemary conley's

solo slim®

"solo slim is a range of healthy, natural food which is low-fat, great tasting and with a long shelf life!"

low-fat **butternut squash, cumin & chilli soup**

a delicious low-fat calorie controlled meal for one

DAY 5

Breakfast ☑
■ 1 yellow Portion Pot® (125ml) fresh orange juice plus 1 red Portion Pot® (40g) Special K cereal served with milk from allowance and 1 tsp sugar

Mid-morning Power Snack ☑
■ 1 Ryvita spread with Marmite and topped with a large sliced tomato

Lunch ☑
■ 1 pouch **Solo Slim® Low-Fat Three Bean Casserole** plus a large salad tossed in fat-free dressing

Mid-afternoon Power Snack ☑
■ 2 satsumas or 2 kiwi fruits

Dinner
■ 1 pouch **Solo Slim® Low-Fat Lamb Hotpot** served with 100g green vegetables of your choice
■ Fresh fruit salad

DAY 6

Breakfast ☑
■ 1 slice wholegrain bread, toasted, topped with 1 yellow Portion Pot® (115g) baked beans
■ 1 piece fresh fruit

Mid-morning Power Snack ☑
■ 75g seedless grapes

Lunch ☑
■ 1 pouch **Solo Slim® Low-Fat Butternut Squash, Cumin and Chilli Soup**
■ 1 slice wholegrain bread, toasted, topped with 30g **Rosemary Conley's low-fat Mature Cheese** and a dash of Worcester sauce, served with a small salad tossed in fat-free dressing

Mid-afternoon Power Snack ☑
■ 1 fresh peach or 150g strawberries

Dinner
■ 1 pouch **Solo Slim® Low-Fat Thai Chicken Curry** plus 25g (dry weight) basmati rice, boiled in water with a vegetable stock cube

DAY 7

Breakfast ☑
- 1 small banana, sliced, mixed with 115g sliced strawberries and 1 × 100g pot yogurt (max. 100 kcal and 5% fat)

Mid-morning Power Snack ☑
- 20g sultanas

Lunch
- 2 slices wholegrain bread spread with very low fat cream cheese (e.g. Philadelphia Extra Light) and topped with 30g smoked salmon served with a small rocket salad

Mid-afternoon Power Snack ☑
- 100g fresh pineapple

Dinner
- 1 pouch **Solo Slim® Low-Fat Three Bean and Chorizo Soup**
- 1 pouch **Solo Slim Low-Fat Moroccan Spiced Chickpea Tagine** plus 100g green vegetables of your choice

> **How to order Solo Slim® meals**
> To order your Stay Young Solo Slim® Healthy Food Box, log on to **www.rosemaryconley.com** or **phone 0870 0507727**. If you have any special dietary requirements, then our mail order department will be happy to help you select your meals. Providing your order is received by 12 noon, from Monday to Thursday, you can be assured that delivery will take place within 24 hours.

GOLDEN RULES FOR SUCCESSFUL WEIGHT LOSS

- Decide on a start day for your diet.
- Remove all tempting foods from the house.
- Decide on your week's menu and write it down.
- Shop accordingly.
- Stick to the diet rules.
- Never skip a meal.
- Do eat your Power Snacks to stave off hunger pangs between meals.

Rosemary Conley's Stay Young Solo Slim® Healthy Food Box

A 7-Day Stay Young Solo Slim® Healthy Food Box contains:

- **9 soups of your choice**
- **8 ready meals of your choice**
- **200g block of Rosemary Conley's 5% fat Mature Cheese**

If you follow the Stay Young Solo Slim® Diet described in this book, here's what you will need to order:

Soups

2 Carrot and Coriander

1 Chunky Vegetable

1 Lentil

1 Tomato

1 Mushroom

1 Minestrone

1 Butternut Squash, Cumin and Chilli

1 Three Bean and Chorizo

Meals (non-vegetarian)

1 Chicken Hotpot

1 Chilli and Rice

1 Beef Casserole

1 Lamb Hotpot

1 Thai Chicken Curry

Meals (vegetarian)

1 Tomato and Vegetable Pasta

1 Three Bean Casserole

1 Moroccan Spiced Chickpea Tagine

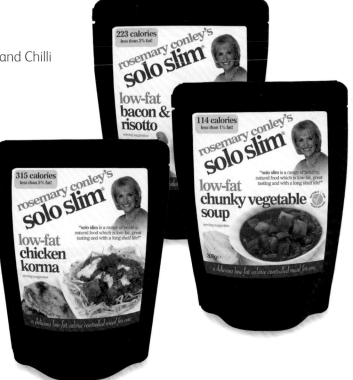

Motivate yourself with a Magic Measure®

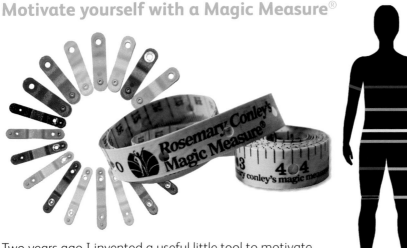

Parts to measure and relevant colour of tags

| Bust / Chest |
| Waist |
| Hips |
| Widest part |
| Left arm |
| Right arm |
| Left thigh |
| Right thigh |
| Left knee |
| Right knee |

Two years ago I invented a useful little tool to motivate dieters in their weight-loss campaign. My Magic Measure® is a tape measure with a hole punched in at each 2.5cm/1 inch marker, through which clips can be fastened to denote your inch-loss progress. There are two sets of colour-coded clips – 'fat' tags and 'slim' tags. Each colour denotes a different part of the body – bust/chest, waist, hips, etc. You clip on the 'fat' tags on at the beginning of your weight-loss campaign, to indicate your starting measurements, and these tags cannot be removed once clipped into position. After the first week, you measure yourself again and clip on the corresponding coloured 'slim' tags at the appropriate new and reduced measurements. As you shed weight you'll easily be able to see how many inches you're losing off each part of your body.

To see a demonstration of how the Magic Measure® works, log on to www.rosemaryconley.tv

One slimmer who found that the Magic Measure® played a key part in motivating her in her weight-loss campaign was Stephanie Hughes. Stephanie was one of my 2011 Slimmers of the Year. She lost an astonishing 145 inches from her body in 12 months, along with 12st 7lb in weight. You can watch Stephanie talking about her weight-and-inch-loss journey on www.rosemaryconley.tv on the Slimmer of the Year 2011 channel.

GOLDEN RULES FOR MEASURING YOURSELF

- Measure yourself at the same time each week.
- Measure yourself in your underwear.
- Use the 'fat' tags to register your 'start' inches.
- Apply the 'slim' tags after one week on the diet and move them along each week.

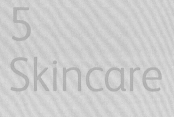

5
Skincare

Frighteningly, our skin begins to deteriorate from the age of 28, but that doesn't mean we can't have healthy looking skin into our 80s. The condition of our skin is determined by many things, including our genes, our exposure to the sun, the food we eat, the amount of alcohol we drink, whether we smoke, work outdoors or even get enough sleep.

Why does our skin wrinkle with age?

The skin is an organ and as such requires constant nourishment and protection. When we're young our skin is kept smooth and plumped up by our natural supply of proteins called elastin and collagen, but as we get older our levels of these proteins reduce and our skin can become slack and hang loosely. In our youth, it's as if we have a layer of 'bubble wrap' under our skin, keeping it plump and firm.

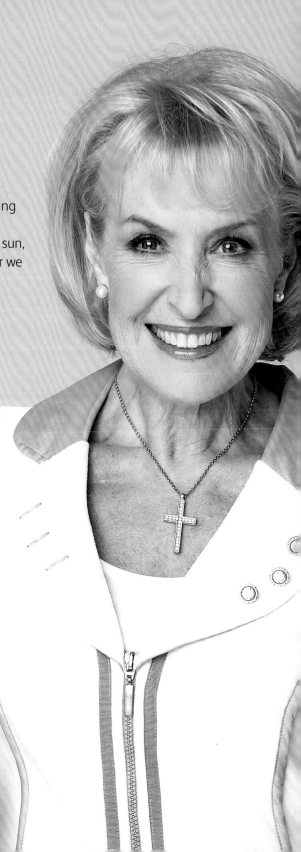

Now imagine that all those pockets of air in new bubble wrap represent our skin cells – buoyant and firm. Over time the bubble wrap becomes less firm and the 'bubbles' lose their strength. That's what happens to our skin when our oestrogen and collagen levels reduce as we age. It loses that lovely layer of buoyancy and appears almost as if it's too big for us. Inevitably, lines and wrinkles begin to appear.

It's the oestrogen in the body that stimulates the production of collagen, the supportive fibrous structure that gives skin its strength and density. Once our oestrogen levels start to decline, the body is unable to produce more oestrogen naturally, so wrinkling and puckering occur, giving the unkind appearance of ageing. At the same time, we lose a lot of subcutaneous fat under our skin as we get older. If we were to look at the back of our hands as we aged, we would see the veins becoming much more prominent, and that's because the layer of fat that used to be under the skin has diminished and the veins become more exposed. It's this loss of fat that causes us to feel the cold much more. Also, our muscles reduce and become smaller and weaker as we get older, both the facial muscles and the muscles in the body. The good news is that we can exercise these muscles effectively and keep them strong to significantly delay the appearance of our advancing years.

The other good news is that we can help slow down the ageing process of our skin by using skincare products that contain 'phytoestrogens', which are plant-based oestrogens. Through advanced technology, phytoestrogens are now available as supplements and taken internally in tablet or capsule form. Phytoestrogens can help skin to retain its thickness and elasticity by encouraging new cells to form and consequently delay the signs of ageing. Since I've been taking Replenish Day-Night Skin Nutrition Supplement I've definitely seen an improvement in my skin, with some of the wrinkles on my cheeks becoming significantly less prominent.

As well as the biological ageing process, the effects of elements in our current-day lifestyle, such as central heating, air conditioning and hard water, can cause skin to become significantly dryer, which makes it look older. Unfortunately, cosmetics applied externally have not been proven to delay the ageing process, but they can certainly help by adding moisture and luminosity to skin so that it looks younger.

When it comes to skincare cosmetics, it's a question of brand preference and your purse. Many cosmetics make some pretty bold claims, promising miracle anti-ageing results. I only know what I like and what suits me, but we're all different.

The golden rule for skincare is that, if you have dry skin, you need to only gently cleanse it, but moisturise it regularly to keep it looking youthful. If you have oily skin, cleansing is key and non-oily moisturisers will help protect it (the good thing about oily skin is that it wrinkles less!). If you have a combination skin – that's dry down the sides and oily down the centre panel (i.e. forehead, nose and chin), you need to treat it accordingly. Cleanse the centre panel with a non-oily product and make sure that any moisturisers or anti-wrinkle creams you use for the central area are non-greasy, otherwise they will encourage open pores and an unattractive appearance. For the drier side panels of your face, treat as dry skin.

Our skin shows what we eat

Another cause of skin ageing is damage from free radicals, which we all have naturally in our body. As we get older, our levels of free radicals increase and it's these free radicals that cause oxidation, which plays a key role in the ageing process. We can, however, minimise this free-radical damage by eating foods high in antioxidants. That's why it's important to eat lots of brightly coloured fruit and vegetables throughout our life, but particularly as we get older.

Anti-ageing creams and supplements are designed to help skin retain its elasticity.

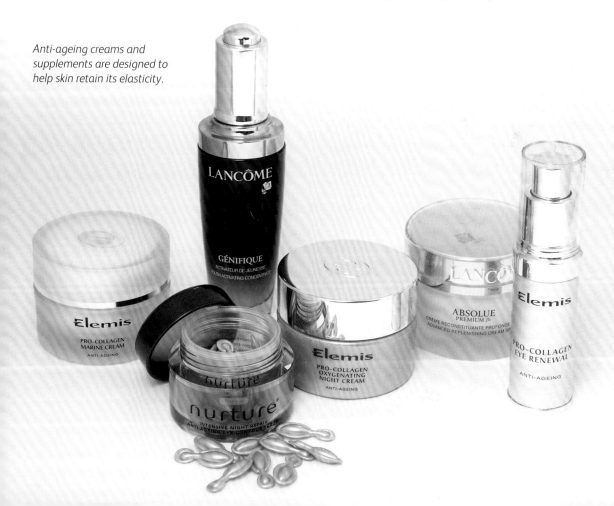

Eating plenty of vegetables helps us to stay young for a variety of reasons. Green leafy vegetables, for instance, are a particularly good source of folate, a B vitamin, which may help to reduce the risk of heart disease by lowering the levels of a substance called homocysteine in the blood. Green leafy vegetables also contain some iron, which is vital for health, though it's not as well absorbed as the iron contained in meat. Many vegetables, including cauliflower, cabbage, sprouts and peas, are rich in vitamin C, which helps us to fight infection. Parsnips are a good source of potassium and may help to control blood pressure. Broccoli is one of the nation's favourite vegetables and the most important source of vitamin K in the diet. Vitamin K is best known for its valuable role in helping blood to clot properly, but it's also important for healthy bones. Red, yellow and other brightly coloured vegetables, such as carrots, beetroot and peppers, are rich in carotenoids, a type of antioxidant that helps the body to fight the free-radical damage caused by pollutants, stress and other factors that are thought to contribute to the ageing process.

The Stay Young Diet in this book is designed to maximise your intake of antioxidants as well as control the calories – it's a stay-young, superfood diet that will help you to feel and look like a new person.

Skincare: Face

Having had very bad eczema as a child, I've suffered from dry skin throughout my life. I apply a moisturising body lotion to my entire body every day after my bath or shower and it certainly helps to keep my skin in reasonable order. After I became pregnant in my late 20s the skin on my face became extremely dry, too, and since then I have been scrupulous in the application of skincare products. Keeping skin nourished and moisturised is fundamental to keeping it looking younger.

I apply these facial skincare products each morning before putting on my makeup: Boots' No 7 Protect & Perfect Intense Beauty Serum, Lancôme's Rénergie anti-wrinkle firming treatment and Dior's Hydra Life pro-youth comfort cream.

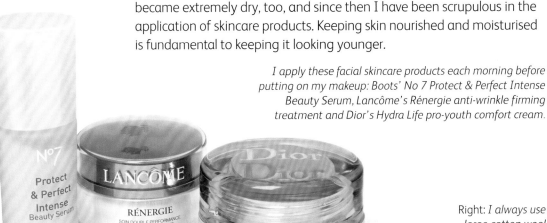

Right: I always use large cotton wool pads dampened with cold water for applying cleansers to remove my facial and eye makeup.

For basic facial skincare, find a cosmetic range that suits your pocket and your skin. By that I mean try out one product to see that you're not allergic to it before investing in a whole range of products. I'm a massive fan of Lancôme skincare products but I also use Boots' No7 Protect and Perfect Intense Beauty Serum, which is lovely.

My daily facial skincare routine

My morning routine involves refreshing my face and neck with a dampened cotton wool pad (I use one of the bigger cotton wool pads and always wet it with cold water and then squeeze it out). Then I apply Boots' No7 Protect and Perfect Intense Beauty Serum, which gives a wonderfully smooth finish. Next I apply an anti-ageing cream, Rénergie by Lancôme, which is good for hydration and I've used it for years. I apply it all over my face and neck, not forgetting my ears, which need nourishing too. I leave it to soak in for, say, 10 minutes before I finally apply a moisturiser to protect my skin from the sun's rays and the elements. Then I apply my makeup – more about that in Chapter 13.

At bedtime I apply a cleansing lotion all over my face and neck with my fingers and use dampened cotton wool pads to remove my makeup. For my eyes, I use an eye makeup removal lotion on a dampened cotton wool pad. I never, ever use dry cotton wool pads or cotton wool balls or tissues on my face as they drag the sensitive skin around the eyes and face. In my opinion, they don't do a very good job and you end up using much more cleansing product than with dampened cotton wool.

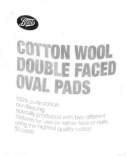

Before I go to bed, I apply a night cream to my face and ears to nourish my skin through the night. It's important to choose an appropriate night cream for your skin type. The beauty consultant at your local department store or high street chemist will advise you as to which one is most suitable for you. I use Nutrix by Lancôme, which is very rich and only suitable for very dry skin types.

About every eight weeks or so I exfoliate my face with a gentle facial exfoliator by Lancôme, called Exfoliance Clarté. If you're not familiar with exfoliators, these are cleansing gels that contain tiny grain-like micro-balls, which you massage onto your face. The slightly rough texture of the exfoliator has the effect of removing any dead cells from the face and stimulating the skin, resulting in a glowing and super-smooth finish.

My best experience of this treatment was at the LaSource health spa resort in Grenada. The beauty therapist gently massaged the slightly grainy lotion onto my face for 30 minutes and then washed it off with warm water. At the end my face had never looked so smooth – and definitely more youthful – and it felt fantastic. There were certainly no dead skin cells left on my face! Since then, I've done it myself, but only for about two to three minutes and only five or six times a year, but I've still enjoyed a visible benefit from it. One word of warning – after you have exfoliated your face, make sure you do not expose the 'bare' skin to the sun without lots of protective sun cream.

Visit www.rosemaryconley.tv to see me discussing skincare with Dr Hilary Jones.

Each evening after cleansing my face and neck and removing my eye makeup, I apply a rich cream to nourish my dry skin. I like to exfoliate my face every eight weeks or so, using Lancôme Exfoliance Clarté.

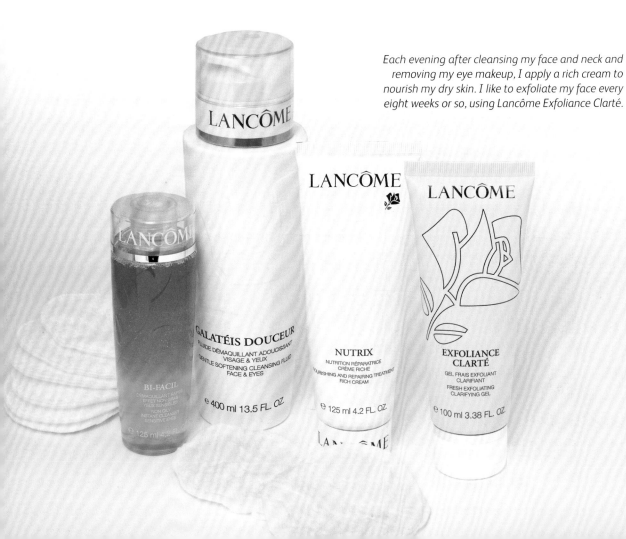

Facials and face masks

There's nothing more relaxing than having a facial, and anyone who visits a health spa will place it near the top of their most enjoyable experiences. A beauty therapist will massage your face, stimulating the circulation around the face and neck area, and it will certainly make you look and feel terrific. Sometimes your treatment will include a face mask, which will deep-feed your face and draw out impurities. Not everyone has the time or the money to experience facials on a regular basis but if you do, go ahead and enjoy it. You can, however, easily and inexpensively treat yourself to a face mask at home. If you suffer from blackheads or spots, you may find this very helpful in reducing the problem.

I used to go to a wonderful beauty therapist who was still working her 'magic' hands well into her 80s, but more recently I only get the chance to have a facial if I'm away and there's a spa where I'm staying, and because I have the time, I treat myself.

GOLDEN RULES FOR THE FACE
- Always use dampened cotton wool to remove makeup.
- Apply anti-ageing cream and moisturiser in the morning.
- Apply a nourishing night cream at night.
- For a super-smooth complexion, use a facial exfoliator every eight weeks.
- Enjoy a facial when you can.

Skincare: Body

The skin on the body can often deteriorate at a faster rate than that on the face because we tend not to look after it as intensely. Even someone who doesn't wear a lot of makeup will almost certainly apply a moisturiser of some kind to their face on a daily basis, but they may not be as motivated to do the same for their body.

While it's true that the body is covered up most of the time and not exposed to pollution and the sun's rays as often as the face, it nevertheless needs to be cared for if it's to stay looking youthful. Again, the ageing effect on the body is down to a lack of moisture as well as the natural reduction in collagen under the surface of the skin.

Sun safety

Excessive exposure to the sun is hugely damaging but we have to weigh up the benefits and costs of acquiring a healthy, moderate tan. Most people say they feel better with a bit of a tan –

I know I do – but unfortunately it comes at a cost. Yes, we can go down the spray tan route but I don't think that looks natural and it makes your skin smell. I've only had it done for recording purposes, such as presenting my fitness DVDs – and I hate it. Mostly, if I have a tan, it's a real one. I wear a moderate sunscreen and I never allow myself to burn. And I always apply loads of body lotion every day, no matter what.

Depending on your body shape, your body will start showing the first signs of ageing in different places. If you're apple-shaped, your legs and arms will be pretty lean anyway and they are likely to get thinner as you get older. Because there's little fat on the arms, they tend to stay in good shape for significantly longer than those of a pear-shaped person. I'm pear-shaped, so my arms and legs are well covered with a layer of fat, which means that my arms started to age quite early – in my early 50s. The first sign was a little puckering in the front of the arm, just above the elbow. As the years have progressed the crinkling has become more obvious if I lean forwards. It's not an attractive look as the fibres of my muscles appear to have become looser and the result is my arms look as if they could do with a good iron! Consequently I wear long sleeves most of the time – but more about that in Chapter 21.

Shrinking the skin through exercise

When we lose weight, our skin obviously needs to contract and we can encourage that by doing very regular aerobic exercise. Aerobic exercise – such as brisk walking, aerobics, running or swimming – makes us breathe more deeply and become slightly breathless. As we do so we force more oxygen into our lungs and our bloodstream, which in turn is circulating around our body and through our muscles. And, because our muscles are working hard in burning fat and being very active during the exercise, this encourages more oxygen to flow closer to the skin, which helps it to be healthier. After all, we perspire through our skin, so we can see that the skin is actively benefiting from the exercise – with the brilliant result that the skin shrinks as we lose weight. This means that if you exercise while you follow a weight-reducing diet, you will have a toned body at the end of your weight-loss campaign.

Skin-firming cream

If you have a lot of weight to lose, particularly if you've been very overweight for a long time, you'll have to take extra care of your skin. My Moisturising Firming Cream can help in that process and many of our Slimmers of the Year have found it extremely effective in helping their skin to shrink back and in minimising stretch marks.

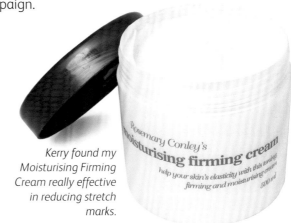

Kerry found my Moisturising Firming Cream really effective in reducing stretch marks.

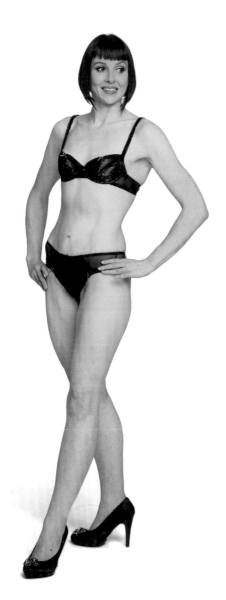

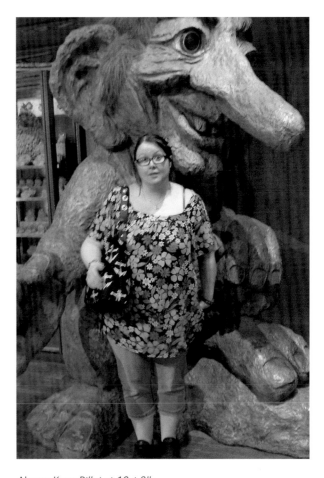

Above: *Kerry Pillai at 19st 8lb.*

Left: *Kerry looking slim and toned after she lost over 10 stone.*

Kerry Pillai lost over 10 stone on my diet at her local Rosemary Conley Diet and Fitness class and went on to appear in my *Real Results Workout* DVD. Her weight loss and dedication to exercise produced a body that you would never believe had been overweight, let alone twice its current weight! Kerry told us that my Moisturising Firming Cream had been extremely effective in reducing the appearance of stretch marks from when she was very overweight.

When I decided to see if we could find a moisturising cream that would be effective, I insisted to the manufacturer that it had to undergo a clinical trial to prove its effectiveness before I would put my name to it. I'm glad to report that the cream passed with flying colours and the evidence I have subsequently witnessed bears that out. I also wanted the cream to be relatively inexpensive and suitable not just for the body but the face as well. My mother-in-law, Jeanne, uses it on her face every night and I use it on my body and have found it helps keep my skin more youthful, particularly the skin on my arms. We have sold thousands and thousands of pots of this brilliant product and our customers love it.

Having said all that, any moisturiser applied to your body is better than none and the action of massaging in the cream is helpful in improving circulation, skin texture and hydration.

GOLDEN RULES FOR BODY SKINCARE

- Apply body lotion all over the body every day without fail.
- Massage the lotion into the skin with strong movements to stimulate circulation.
- Exfoliate your body every three months to remove dead skin cells and keep skin looking smooth and youthful.

Always choose skincare products that suit your skin type. Left to right: Eucerin Intensive Treatment Lotion, Aveeno Moisturising Creamy Oil, Aveeno Daily Moisturising Lotion and Aveeno Skin Relief Moisturising Lotion – all great products for dry skin.

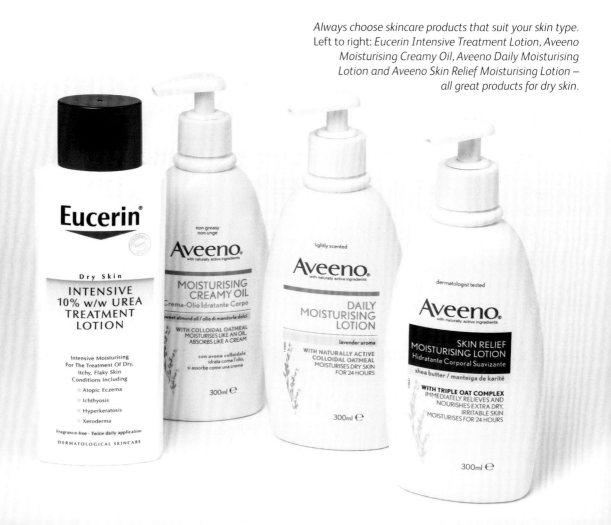

Skincare: Feet

Having squeezed my very small (size 3) feet into high heels for the last 50 years, it's not surprising that my feet are not my best feature. They have been treated with little respect. For me, my feet were best covered up and ignored, that is until I stood on a stone and it cut the skin under one of my feet. As I sat on the floor, contorting into an advanced lotus position to examine the cut, I had a horrible shock. The soles of my feet looked like turtle skin! I was shocked. My feet looked like they should have belonged to someone who had received a telegram from the Queen!

My chiropodist had mentioned foot cream before, but I'd not bothered with it. It all seemed a bit unnecessary. How wrong I was! I purchased some CCS Foot Care Cream from Boots and started applying it lovingly to my turtle-skin feet. After a while, not only did they look as though they were now the same age as me instead of 40 years older, my feet *felt* so much better. They didn't get so tired, they didn't ache and I stopped getting dry skin on my soles. It was a transforming experience and I am now a total advocate of foot cream. It's not expensive, it lasts for ages and makes my feet now look as if they belong to a human rather than an alien!

For all the fact that I've abused my feet by wearing high heels since I was 15, I have every intention of carrying on doing so. I wear high heels most of the time, not just because I'm so short but because I feel more elegant when I do. They help to keep my ankles slim and make my legs look longer. I have no trouble walking in flat shoes and do so every day when I walk the dogs or teach exercise.

However, one of the problems of getting older is that the protective fatty pad on the ball of the foot gets thinner. Consequently, the balls of my feet do get a bit sore when I've been standing in high heels for most of the day. Fortunately, I've made a brilliant discovery: Insolia Insert (available from www.simplyfeet.co.uk). You put these clever little gel pads under your heel and insole rather than under the ball of the foot. They are very effective in transferring the weight from the ball of the foot to the heel to make high-heel wearing infinitely more comfortable.

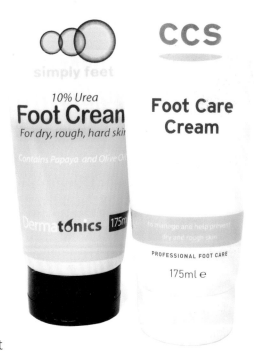

I love both of these: Simply Feet 10% Urea Foot Cream and CCS Foot Care Cream.

Marks and Spencer has cleverly incorporated Insolia Inserts into many of its fashion shoes, making them ultra-comfortable.

A pedicure makes a special treat for feet but you can also do this yourself at home. Set aside half an hour once a week to soak your feet in a bowl of warm water with a couple of drops of oil added to soften the skin. Then use a cotton bud to gently ease back the cuticles. Next, cut nails straight across, using clippers or scissors. Never cut down at the sides as this can cause ingrown toenails. Finally, apply foot cream over your feet.

Keep hard skin at bay by rubbing it gently with a pumice stone in the morning when you shower or take a bath. Once a week, use a foot file on clean, dry skin. Don't overdo it, though, as too much filing can leave skin feeling sore and uncomfortable to walk on.

Any foot problems should be dealt with by a podiatrist, who will be able to treat corns and calluses, seriously cracked heels, impacted nails, fungal infections and verrucas. Don't try to tackle these yourself at home. Even if you're not experiencing any problems it's a good idea to visit a podiatrist every three to six months for an overhaul of your feet. Once you've had your feet cared for professionally, you can maintain the good results at home.

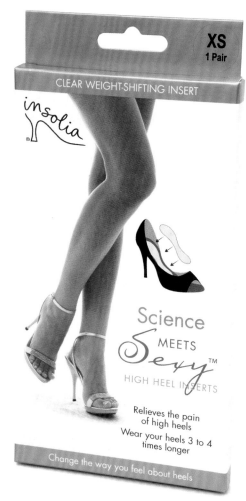

I find these gel pads brilliant for reducing the discomfort caused by wearing high heels.

GOLDEN RULES FOR FEET

- Apply foot cream to your feet daily after your shower or bath.
- Use a pumice stone on hard skin when you shower or take a bath.
- Visit a podiatrist every three to six months.
- Cut your toenails regularly.
- Have an occasional pedicure.
- If you wear high heels, use Insolia Inserts in your shoes.

Skincare: Hands

I think we learn a lot of habits from our mothers, and looking after our hands and applying hand cream every time we've had our hands in water is a habit that we're either brought up with or we're not. My mother didn't have this habit and neither did I, and it's something I deeply regret. Having suffered with chronic eczema as a very young child and then into adulthood, my hands have suffered under endless steroid treatments and the skin is thin and older-looking than it should be. I suppose, like my feet, I'd 'written-off' my hands as being unattractive because of their dryness and, stupidly, I've not kept them moisturised with hand cream when I should have. As a result, my hands are not my best feature, though I am now trying to make up for past neglect by applying hand cream as often as possible, wearing rubber gloves to do the washing up and giving them a good soaking of hand cream just before I go to bed so that they can absorb it through the night.

On top of this, we lose a lot of subcutaneous fat under the skin as we get older – the veins at the back of our hands become more prominent, not because the veins have got bigger, but because there's not enough fat and collagen underneath the skin to keep the skin plumped up. This is why we feel the cold more and why we bruise more easily as we age – there's no longer the insulation that used to be there.

Fortunately, I have strong nails, which helps the appearance of my hands, and I don't have arthritic joints, for which I am grateful. Age spots have not appeared too prolifically yet, but no doubt they will in time! If you already have age spots, why not try one of the products that's designed to minimise them. Healthspan Nurture has a product called Replenish Intensive Pigmentation Reducing Complex, which has received good reports and is said to be very effective.

Healthspan Nurture's Replenish Intensive Pigmentation Reducing Complex helps to minimise age spots. Apply hand cream regularly, particularly at night, to keep hands looking younger.

As my hands aren't one of my better features I don't draw attention to them by wearing bright nail polish. Occasionally I wear a clear varnish or, for a special occasion, French nail polish, which highlights the nail tips in white. I keep my nails tidy and in shape with an emery board and never use a metal file.

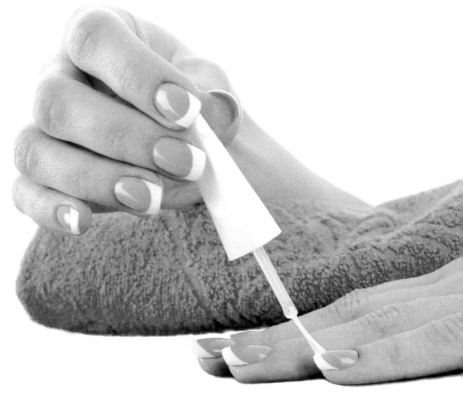

I'm not a fan of acrylic nails as they can damage the nail bed, but they can provide a lifeline if you need to repair a nail before an important occasion when you want your nails to look perfect. If you prefer to use coloured nail varnish, always apply a clear base coat first to protect your nails, and try to leave your nails varnish-free for one day a week to prevent long-term discolouration.

GOLDEN RULES FOR HANDS
- Always wear rubber gloves for washing up.
- Apply hand cream whenever possible, particularly last thing at night.
- Keep nails manicured.
- Use an emery board rather than a metal file to file nails.

6
Stay Young
facial exercise
and toning

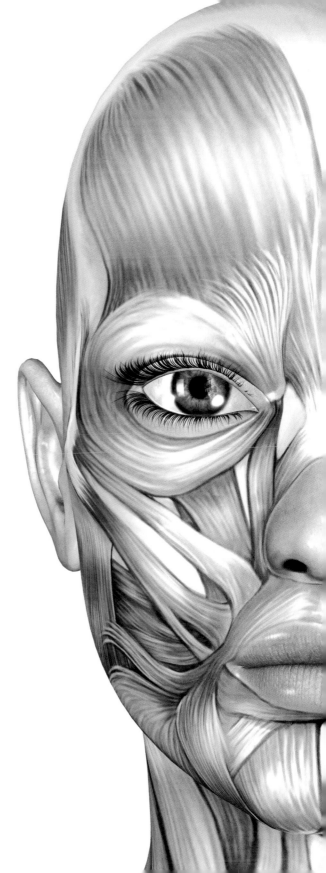

The face is constructed of a vast network of muscles that give it its shape and features. As we become older our facial muscles can reduce dramatically and our appearance can change. Sometimes that change can be good, and I prefer the shape and definition of my face now I'm in my 60s than when I was younger.

About seven years ago I was sent a gadget to try out called Facial-Flex®. It was created by a surgeon to help patients with facial burns exercise their faces in an attempt to rebuild their damaged features. But then something happened that he hadn't expected. Because the physiotherapists were demonstrating the device regularly, they began to show signs of improved facial toning and lifting, which resulted in the physiotherapists all looking much younger! Consequently, it was decided to manufacture Facial-Flex® as a cosmetic anti-ageing device and I'm a huge fan. I use it every day for around two minutes twice a day and it has had a dramatic effect in the strengthening and retention of the muscles around my mouth, jawline, chin and chest.

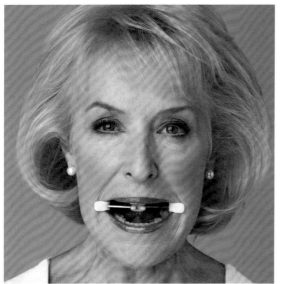
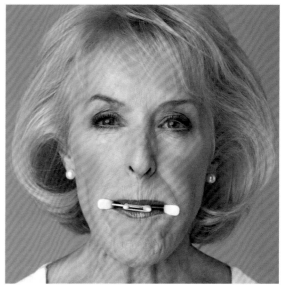

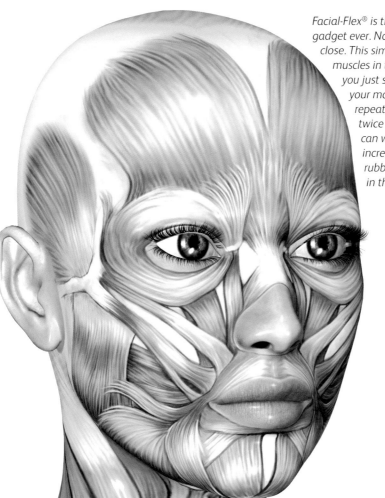

Facial-Flex® is the most effective face-toning gadget ever. Nothing else I've tried comes even close. This simple tool, which works about 30 muscles in the face and neck, is easy to use – you just squeeze the two ends together in your mouth then release it – and you repeat the action for just two minutes twice a day. For even better results, you can work the muscles harder by increasing the strength of the little rubber bands that provide the resistance in the centre of the Facial-Flex®.

Facial-Flex® works the facial muscles in the same way that a toning band works the muscles of the body. Quite simply, the Facial-Flex® device is placed between the two corners of the mouth and is held together in the centre by a small rubber band. As you squeeze the two ends of the device inwards (together), it automatically stretches the rubber band, offering 'resistance' and making the facial muscles work harder. Just by squeezing and releasing the tension in your mouth you will activate up to 30 different facial muscles and make them work harder. Over time, those muscles will become stronger and slightly bigger, reversing the shrinkage of the lips and the surrounding area to give a fuller, plumper lip appearance and a lifting of the jawline, toning up a double chin, the neck and even down to the chest.

I was so impressed by the product that we are now the sole distributors of Facial-Flex® in the UK, but my instructions for its use vary slightly after fine-tuning its use for myself. The tiny rubber bands that enable Facial-Flex® to work come in three strengths – 1, 2 and 3. A supply of No 1 bands comes with the device, with the recommendation that one should change the bands weekly to maintain their strength and power. As you become stronger around the mouth, you can increase your band strength.

As a fitness professional, I understand that to encourage muscles to become bigger and stronger we need to increase the 'load' so that the muscles work harder. Accordingly, I now use two No 3 bands for my facial workout and, because they're so strong, I only need to change the bands every couple of months or so, making it more economical too. I use my Facial-Flex® without fail every day for around 60 contractions – in the morning and before I go to bed. It's really effective in toning up the facial muscles from the cheeks down. But as it only works on the muscles of the lower face, Facial-Flex® will not help with crow's feet or lines around the eyes.

While the device isn't cheap, it's of high quality and will last for years (I'm still using my original one), and the bands are inexpensive to replace.

In 2010, Facial-Flex® was given a top beauty award in France – Victoire de la Beauté 2010/2011 – so you don't have to just take my word for it that it really is effective.

Facial-Flex® is available from www.rosemaryconley.com

GOLDEN RULES FOR FACIAL EXERCISES

- Use your Facial-Flex® every day without fail.
- Use as strong a band as possible.
- Double-up on bands to offer greater resistance.
- Change bands regularly to maximise strength.

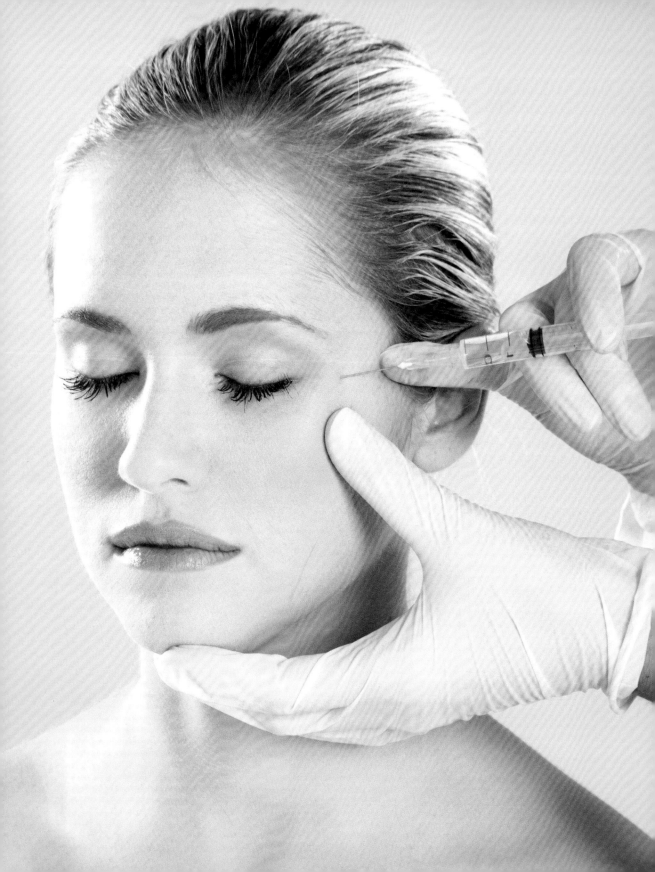

7
Cosmetic surgery, Botox, fillers and the like

I can't give you any insight into cosmetic surgery as I've never had it. I've considered it but decided it would be too risky and, in any event, once you start, where do you stop?

About eight years ago I tried Isolagen treatment, where a piece of skin is taken from behind your ear and sent to a laboratory. Stem cells are grown from the skin sample and then injected into your face to help plump up the lines around your eyes and elsewhere. The advantage of this treatment is that the cells being injected into your face are your own and they continue the characteristics of your skin at the age the sample was extracted. So, in theory, if your skin sample was taken when you were 50, you could have those skin cells (aged 50) injected into your face even when you were 80! It sounds a great idea.

I had the treatment a couple of times quite successfully, but apparently it only works in around 60 per cent of cases. Not surprisingly, many patients were very disappointed and, before long, Isolagen was no more in the UK. The treatment wasn't cheap and it only worked for a limited period of time so, all in all, I should have saved my money.

There are other 'fillers' available and some people find them very effective but the thought of putting a needle *into and under* my wrinkles to inject the 'filler' sounds unbelievably painful to me!

I have, however, experimented with Botox with mixed results. I had it on my forehead, but the flesh above my eyelids became baggy, which was not attractive. It can also have the effect of making you look distinctly startled, which, in my opinion, is not a good look either. So now, about once a year, I just have Botox injected into my laughter lines at the sides of my eyes. I don't look dramatically different for having the treatment, but it just softens those lines and stops them becoming too deep and ingrained. I don't have anything else done.

There are a variety of non-surgical treatments available on the market and if you want to find out more, you can contact one of the growing number of clinics for more information. But it's important to remember that all non-surgical interventions have only a temporary effect, they are quite expensive and their results are limited.

Personally, I think Facial-Flex® is the most inexpensive, incredibly effective aid to keeping the lower half of your face looking naturally toned. The difference it has made to my face is dramatic. However, as it doesn't work the muscles above your cheeks, if you want to minimise the lines around your outer eye area, Botox is probably worth a try. It lasts for about six months and isn't too painful.

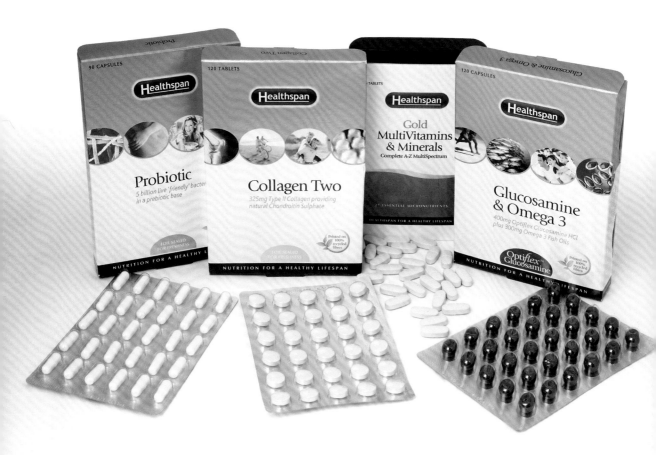

8
Nutritional supplements

We often see advertisements for nutritional supplements that promise to help reverse the signs of ageing and the claims made by the manufacturers are certainly enticing.

Many doctors will tell you there's no clinical evidence to show that most supplements will help. So we're left to make our own choices and decisions.

I take several supplements every day. I take a combined glucosamine and omega 3 supplement daily to help protect my joints into the future. Because I don't eat enough oily fish in my diet, which we need to keep the heart healthy, the omega 3 also helps protect against heart disease. I also take two Type II collagen supplements a day, which helps protect joint cartilage. This type of collagen helps maintain the connective tissue that lines the surface of joints to keep them supple and healthy. When this cartilage degenerates, it can lead to painful rubbing of bone on bone in the joints.

After the age of 60, the body become less efficient at processing food, so I take a probiotic each day to help maintain the levels of good bacteria in my gut. As this also helps get rid of bloating I think it helps to keep my tummy flatter.

I also take a multivitamin tablet daily and I think everyone should do so, just as an insurance policy to ensure we are getting all the necessary micronutrients that are important to health, whether or not we are dieting.

Over the last year or so, I've been taking Replenish Day-Night Skin Supplement from Healthspan Nurture. I take one 'daytime' tablet in the morning and one 'nighttime' capsule before I go to bed. Healthspan claims that this phytoestrogen supplement feeds and replenishes the skin from deep below the skin's surface where traditional creams cannot reach. Does it work? I think it does as I have seen a noticeable difference in my face, with the 'curtain' lines that occur on women's cheeks as they get older becoming significantly less noticeable.

All the above supplements are available from Healthspan (www.healthspan.co.uk) or Healthspan Nurture (www.nurtureskincare.co.uk).

9
Haircare

Our hair undergoes many changes as we age, particularly after the menopause. The reduction in our hormones can affect the condition of our hair, often making it dryer and duller, with reduced elasticity and a change in colour as grey hairs gradually appear. It's also likely that our hair will become thinner, particularly if thinning hair runs in the family. Hair that has a dry texture is likely to snap more easily, but with regular haircare, there's a lot we can do to help our hair.

Grey hair can look stunning and some women find they go grey in their 20s. My mother-in-law, Jeanne, went grey in her 40s and her wonderful grey hair suits her beautifully. But most women will start seeing just the odd grey hair in their 30s and then gradually the evidence of grey will become greater as the years pass by. Some women decide to cover their grey hair with a colour, which takes time and money, while others allow it to become grey gradually and naturally. It's a matter of personal choice.

My hair is naturally a little darker than the blonde you are used to seeing me with. Blonde hair suits me better than my natural colour, so I've had highlights put in my hair for years and grey hairs aren't really an issue for me. They are probably there but camouflaged by my colour. I get the odd grey eyebrow hair, which I hastily pluck out, as I'm not ready to go grey yet!

Shampooing and conditioning

As with our skin, we need to add extra moisture to our hair as we get older to aid hydration and general condition, so care should be taken to select the right shampoo and conditioner.

I have very fine hair and not a huge amount of it, but I always use a volumising shampoo followed by a volumising conditioner. I then use Volumize Leave-in Conditioner mousse and a product called Perfect Hair, both by System Professional at Wella, to give my hair more body. So-called 'volumising' products help to plump up the hair, enabling it to be lifted and styled more easily. Volumising shampoos tend to be 'lighter' than regular shampoos, which can be too heavy for fine mature hair. If you saw my hair in its natural state, you wouldn't believe that I could have a head of hair that looks relatively normal. What I've found, though, is that I don't need to wash my hair as frequently as it's become less greasy now I'm older. That's a great bonus!

If you're fortunate enough to have coarser hair, a 'heavier' shampoo can work perfectly, but it could make very fine hair look lifeless.

Colouring and adding shine and lustre

Hair continues to grow at the same rate whatever our age but, sadly, we may see our hair thinning a little on top as we get older. Adding colour to our hair can give the illusion of thicker hair and there are lots of different types of colour to choose from.

Colouring agents called 'quasi' colours are considered the most suitable for maturing hair as they contain peroxide but no ammonia. This type of colouring product covers grey hairs very effectively, and as they are semi-permanent they wash out over a period of weeks but avoid the need to touch up the roots, as you would do when using a permanent colouring agent.

A permanent colour may be your preferred choice, but it will look much more natural if you use a mixture of colours. Having strands of hair treated with different colours and placed in foils during the treatment gives a very natural-looking head of hair that doesn't look dyed.

If you want to colour your hair, I strongly suggest you find a reputable salon with specialist colourists who colour clients' hair all day and every day. They will have the skill and experience to advise you appropriately for your hair. I go to KH Hair Salon in Leicester and have done so for 39 years. My colourist, Sharon, does a brilliant job in making my lightened hair look natural all the time.

Solutions for problem hair

If you find your hair looking dull and lifeless, you can treat yourself to a product specifically designed to add shine and lustre, but, remember, what you eat will be reflected in your hair. Eat a healthy diet and your hair will benefit enormously. You can also try an anti-ageing conditioning hair treatment such as Healthspan Nurture's hair treatment, which comes in small capsules. Each capsule contains a serum composed of a blend of silicones, keratin amino acids, apricot kernel oil and antioxidant vitamins C and E, which has been successfully trialled and proven to help improve hair condition and make

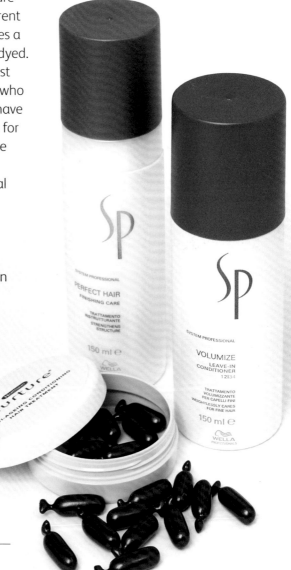

hair more manageable and shiny. Just wash and condition your hair in the usual way, then open the capsule by twisting off the end, squeeze the serum on to your fingertips and apply to towel-dried hair. I've only recently started using this product and I really like it. It definitely makes my hair less flyaway without making it heavy.

If you choose to maintain your grey hair, it can appear a little yellow sometimes, which is not particularly attractive. To help counter this you can use a purple shampoo that simply reduces the yellowness and gives a beautifully rich grey colour. I occasionally use this if my hair goes a bit yellow in the summer sunshine, though usually I try to wear a cap or hat to protect it from becoming overly bleached in the sun. As my hair is coloured, it goes very light in the sun – too much so sometimes – and using a purple shampoo neutralises the tone and makes my hair look less yellow.

Styling

Having discovered the right shampoo, conditioner, special styling products and your preferred colour, the next step is choosing the best style for your hair and lifestyle. Some folk are extremely adept at using hot-air styling brushes, tongs, straighteners, and so on, but others aren't. If you don't want to be bothered with styling your hair, then a wash-and-go, low-maintenance style is best. Some women simply go to the hairdressers once a week to have their hair 'done' and that's it until the next week. It's a very individual thing.

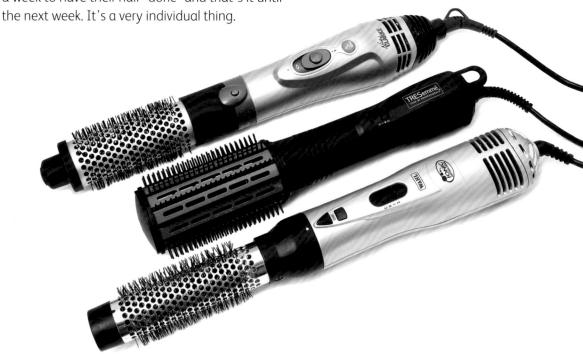

One of the benefits of a higher-maintenance hairstyle is that you will be helping your arms and shoulders to become more flexible by regularly styling your hair with your hands above and behind your head! By holding the hot-air brush, back-combing your hair and so on you are using the muscles and extending the range of movement in your upper body brilliantly.

Back-combing is very effective in adding volume to hair and keeping a style in place. The danger is that if the style is too rigid you can end up looking as though you are wearing a hat and that isn't a youthful look! Use back-combing only to add a little volume and then apply a light hairspray to hold it in place. Your hair should still move a little.

When I was a little girl, my mother, who was very enterprising, created a product called a 'beauty cap', which consisted of a ruched nylon band with ribbons on each end. The idea in the 1950s was to place the beauty cap over your curlers when you went to bed, to make you look more glamorous! Well, Mother managed to manufacture the beauty caps locally with the help of her fellow members of the WI, who were more than willing to earn a little extra towards the housekeeping. Mother even sold the beauty caps through Harrods! As a little girl I was employed – very happily I might add – with my friend Elizabeth to pack the beauty caps in cellophane packets for 3d a dozen!

Thankfully, nobody sleeps in rollers any more and we have endless electrical gadgets to help us curl, crimp, straighten and style our hair in any fashion we like. I use a blow-air brush to give a general style, followed by piece-by-piece curling my hair with straighteners – I realise that sounds a bit back to front, but hair

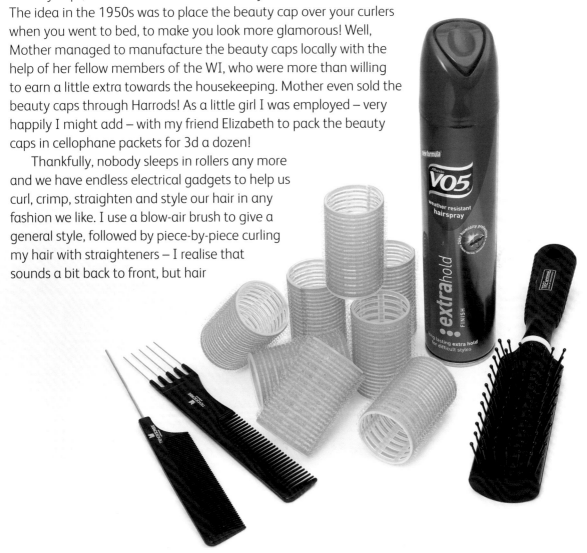

straighteners can be used to curl hair incredibly effectively as well as straighten it too. The ceramic plates that provide the heat get extremely hot so you will need to spray a thermal hair protector product onto your hair to stop your hair becoming over-dry or brittle. These aren't cheap, but they last a long time and are worth the investment to protect your hair. I use Sebastian Shine Define contouring thermal shield to protect mine. If you have very fine hair you may find that using straighteners is too harsh on your hair, in which case the key is to run the straighteners over your hair quite swiftly so they don't scorch it.

To curl your hair, just place the very hot ends of the straighteners at the root of a small section of hair and slide the straighteners through your hair in a half-moon shape, twisting your wrist, to create a curl. You can do ringlet-type curls, too, if you roll the hair around as you slide the appliance along your hair more slowly, but that's more complicated. Your hairstylist should be able to show you how to do it.

Of course, if you have frizzy or curly hair that you prefer to be straight, you simply slide the straighteners down the length of your hair and it will miraculously straighten. Again, use the protective spray to keep your hair healthy.

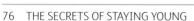

As I curl each section of hair I roll my hair around Velcro rollers (a brilliant invention as they just stick, without the need for pins or clips). This keeps the curled hair out the way while I continue to curl the rest of my hair. It sounds like a real performance but I can do it in a matter of four to five minutes. Once the curlers are in, I apply my makeup, then five minutes later I whisk out the curlers and style my hair. I back-comb it all over and then gradually style it into shape with the end of a tail comb, making sure I look at the back of my head in a mirror. I certainly don't want to go out resembling a bird's nest or Mrs Slocombe! When I'm happy that it looks OK, I spray it with Alberto VO5 Hairspray Extra Firm Hold, which I find is the best product for the job.

If you want a more natural style and don't want to use electrical curling/straightening appliances on your hair, you can blow-dry your hair into your chosen style with a regular hairdryer. To add extra volume, hang your head upside down while drying. This gives extra lift as you will be drying the roots with the hair away from the scalp. You can also spray your hair with hairspray when your head is upside down to add volume, too, and then just encourage your hair into your normal style when you stand up normally again. This is particularly helpful for longer styles as it helps long hair look fuller and avoids that 'stuck to the scalp' look.

Few older women look good with long hair worn loose, but up-styled it can look flattering and elegant. My mother-in-law, Jeanne, wears her hair up all the time and always looks wonderful. She styles it herself, back-combing it and curling it round into a French pleat that looks beautiful every day. I'm sure all that regular arm-lifting helps her to stay active and flexible.

GOLDEN RULES FOR HAIRCARE

- Find a hair salon that will take good care of your hair.
- Choose a style that flatters your face.
- Choose a style that you can manage yourself.
- Decide whether you will stick with the grey or commit to colouring your hair.
- Find haircare products that suit your hair.

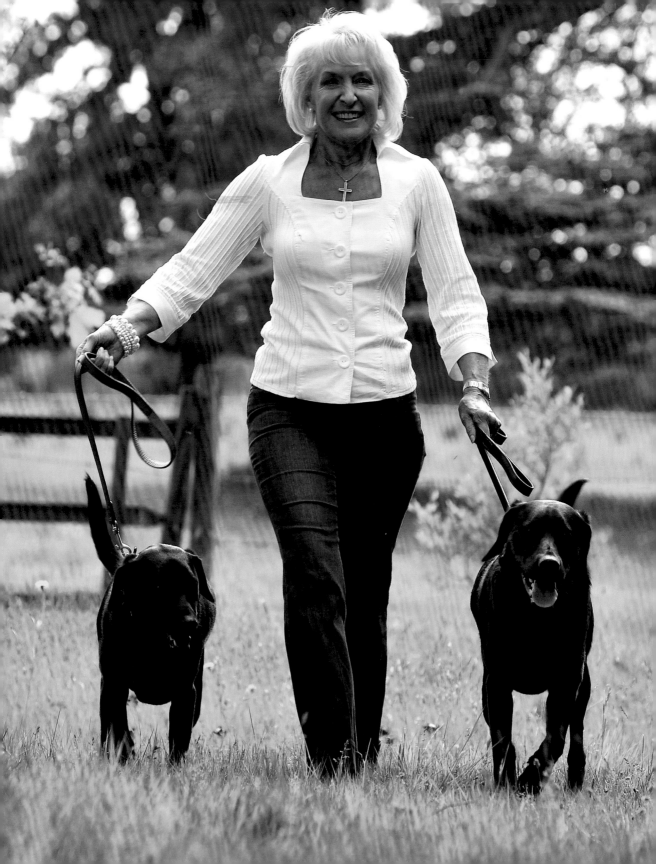

10 Staying healthy into old age

Heart disease, high blood pressure, stroke, high cholesterol, Type 2 diabetes and some cancers are all conditions and illnesses that can devastate our lives. But we have the power to adapt our lifestyles to prevent most of these life-threatening conditions.

By eating a healthy low-fat diet, exercising regularly, keeping – or getting – our weight to a healthy level, drinking alcohol moderately and avoiding smoking, we can drastically reduce our risk of all these conditions.

Dementia is another real worry as we get older. I remember once forgetting where I'd parked my car when I came out of the hairdressers. I went to where I thought I'd left it and it wasn't there. It was one of those moments when I thought, 'This is it! I'm getting Alzheimer's – really!' I was just approaching my 53rd birthday at the time and I was convinced this was the beginning of the end. Fortunately, I found my car two streets away – where I then remembered leaving it – and I waited for more memory lapses to emerge. Fortunately, apart from the usual silly things that are forgotten in a busy life, I'm glad to report that there have been no further frightening lapses of memory and I put down the 'lost car' situation to my being preoccupied with a stressful situation that was going on in my life at that time.

Having high blood pressure and high cholesterol in middle age can seriously increase the risk of developing dementia. High cholesterol and blood pressure can reduce the circulation of nutrients from our food and oxygen to the brain, which, if allowed to persist, can have a significant effect on our mental function. But a low-fat diet rich in green leafy vegetables, oily fish and the occasional glass of red wine can significantly lower our chances of developing dementia, and some studies have shown that this type of Mediterranean diet can reduce the risk by up to 40 per cent.

It's important to have a health check periodically and your GP will be able to check your blood pressure and weight very easily. If you are able to, it's a good idea to have a full medical, although these are often taken by the 'worried well'. However, we are very fortunate that in the UK our NHS health screening is extremely good, particularly for the over-50s and 60s. Breast, cervical and bowel screening are available to us free of charge and are well worth accepting, as early diagnosis could save your life.

We can help to reduce our cholesterol levels by eating a low-fat diet and by including more fibre in our diet, particularly foods with soluble fibre, such as porridge oats, lentils, beans and nuts

– go easy on the nuts, though, if you're trying to lose weight. Fruit and vegetables are also rich in soluble fibre and contain valuable antioxidants. Among their many other benefits, antioxidants stop cholesterol from creating fatty plaques that 'fur up' our arteries. Aerobic exercise reduces our levels of 'bad' cholesterol and increases our 'good' cholesterol and this is perfect for our health. As we get older it is even more important to have our cholesterol levels checked as too high a level can lead to a heart attack or stroke.

Statins are one of the most commonly prescribed medications for people with high cholesterol. They are very effective in reducing cholesterol levels, and therefore reducing the risk of coronary heart disease and strokes. However, one of the common side effects of statins is a feeling of intense fatigue and lethargy and this is partly as a result of a reduction – by as much as 40 per cent – in the amount of the naturally occuring co-enzyme Q10 in the body. There is good evidence that taking a co-enzyme Q10 supplement can offset much of the fatigue that many people experience and, as this is a very safe treatment, it is often recommended by heart specialists and GPs alike when people suffer from the side effects of statins.

Healthy bones

Then there are our bones, of course. The brittle bone disease osteoporosis is a real worry for many older women, although men can suffer from it too. Each bone in the body is a living organ and it's estimated that bones completely renew and replace themselves every seven to ten years. By the age of 30 we achieve our peak bone mass and then, after we reach 40, we begin to lose bone mass – fortunately at a fairly slow rate – as we get older. However, some factors, such as a diet deficient in good nutrition, a lack of exercise, hormonal decline due to the menopause, or – and this is the big one – a family history of osteoporosis, can cause our bones to deteriorate significantly and at a faster rate, leading to osteoporosis and a real risk of breakages.

The good news is there's a lot we can do to help protect the health and strength of our bones. HRT and weight-bearing exercise such as brisk walking and jogging, dancing and aerobics, skipping or even little half-jumps, say about 20, where the heels land heavily, will all stimulate bone density. In addition, any exercise that challenges our muscles, for instance conditioning exercises using light weights or a resistance band, will also help to strengthen bones, as it is the pull of the muscle across the bone that stimulates bone growth and strength.

However, if you already have osteoporosis, it's important not to do high-impact activities (activities where both feet are off the ground at the same time) such as jogging or running, as this will put too much strain on your bones. Low-impact exercise such as walking or gentle aerobics is ideal.

Swimming and cycling are non-impact activities and although they are effective cardiovascular activities, they won't be as effective in strengthening your bones as high- or low-impact forms of exercise.

Another great benefit of exercising regularly is that it helps our sense of balance, coordination and confidence, which reduces our risk of having a fall.

Calcium and vitamins D and K are important for bone health. Calcium is found in dairy products such as milk, yogurts and cheese and the calcium content is not reduced in low-fat versions of these foods. It's precisely for this reason that I include 450ml (¾ pint) of milk in all my diet plans. Calcium is also found in green leafy vegetables and canned fish, particularly sardines. If you're unable to take dairy foods, it will be necessary for you to take a calcium supplement. If you are over 50, you should be taking 700mg of calcium every day.

Vitamin D is essential to help the absorption and retention of the calcium in your diet. The main source of vitamin D is sunlight, and other sources include oily fish, cod liver oil, dairy products and liver.

Vitamin K, also important for bone health, can be found in green leafy vegetables, soya beans, olive oil and margarine. If you're trying to lose weight and you don't want to have olive oil, margarine and cod liver oil because of the fat calories they contain, a daily vitamin K supplement will be your best option to ensure you are doing everything you can to protect your bones and keep them healthy and strong.

If you have a history of osteoporosis in your family, you need to take preventative action. Broken bones are no joke as you get older and anything you can do now to prevent that happening has to be worth the effort.

I presume my bones are strong because of my consistent physical activity over the years and also now because I take HRT, which can help prevent brittle bones, but I did break both my wrists, on two separate occasions, when I was in my 40s. Fortunately, I know my bones are stronger now as I've fallen over many times when ice-skating, without any drastic consequences!

Joints

As we get older we have to expect the odd aching joint now and again. When we are younger, our joints move easily and the synovial fluid that 'oils' them is plentiful. As we age, the synovial fluid is less plentiful and we can get out of the car after a long journey and feel quite 'creaky'! Another cause of aching joints can be the degeneration of the cartilage between joints (cartilage is the flexible rubbery substance in our joints that supports and protects bones), which can lead to the very painful situation of bone rubbing against bone. So what can we do to help prevent this happening to us?

Losing weight is the first priority, as carrying 'excess baggage' puts enormous strain on our joints with a real risk of increased and earlier damage to them.

Next, it's exercise. Different types of exercise and activities can have a significant and valuable effect on strengthening our muscles and the ligaments that hold the skeleton together. Using the Wii Fit, attending a fitness class, exercising to a fitness DVD or participating in a sport regularly will help maintain your muscle strength and keep you and your bones fitter for longer.

Choose a diet rich in calcium and vitamin D and K to help your bones and make sure you spend some time outside in the open air and sunshine to boost your vitamin D levels. Also, if you suffer from inflammation of the joints, try eating foods rich in omega 3 oils (or take a supplement) to reduce the inflammation.

Glucosamine has been widely recognised as being a real help in keeping cartilage healthy and reducing joint damage, as well as improving pain and stiffness as a result of arthritis. As I mentioned earlier, I take a combined glucosamine and omega 3 supplement daily to help keep mine from deteriorating. So far I'm doing fine and I'm hoping it stays that way.

The latest kid on the block in nutritional supplements to help joints is Litozin. Litozin uses just one ingredient – rose hip powder – and, unlike other over-the-counter joint pain relievers, it relies on this one substance to treat the joint pain. The rose hip in Litozin is dried via a patented process and is said to have high levels of GOPO (glycoside of monoglyscerol and diglycerol). This is a clinically tested ingredient that in studies has shown to reduce joint pain more successfully than other standard painkillers. In one study, GOPO reduced pain in 82 per cent of users in just three weeks. There are no known side effects associated with Litozin and the product is 100 per cent natural and suitable for vegetarians. Litozin is produced and sold by Lanes Health (www.laneshealth.com) but is available in some retail stores on the high street.

If you find your health suffering, don't put it down to just getting older. Go to see your doctor sooner rather than later to see if something can be done. We have the best medicines and professional help available to us. We should use them and benefit from it and then we'll live longer.

Log on to www.rosemaryconley.tv to learn more about health issues from Dr Hilary Jones.

11
The psychology of ageing

Hardly a week goes by without some study or report being published announcing that older folk with a positive attitude will live longer, but as weight is harder to shift and exercise can be more challenging, what's the answer to getting our heads around the fact that we're getting older?

Professor Raj Persaud is an internationally renowned psychologist and psychiatrist. He writes for my magazine and regularly appears on our web TV channel to discuss the psychology of weight loss and a healthy lifestyle. I asked him his views on the subject of ageing.

Raj explained that research evidence on dementia is very interesting. If we want to stave off dementia, we need to stay physically fit. So the most important thing we can do as we get older is to take plenty of exercise. Taking up new hobbies and learning new activities is crucial for all sorts of reasons but it's also particularly valuable for reducing our risk of dementia. The brain builds new nerve cells with every new thing we take up, so as we get older learning new skills is brilliant for the brain. Why not take up a sport or physical activity that you have not tried before? Never think it's too late or not the right time in your life – it's precisely the right time.

Personally, I'd never ice-skated in my life until I was asked in 2006 to audition for ITV1's *Dancing on Ice*. Before the audition I signed up for a few lessons at Nottingham Ice Centre and it was one of the hardest skills I have ever attempted. I wasn't selected for the programme but I continued with the occasional lesson. After a two-year break from the ice while I completed two more fitness DVDs – I didn't dare risk breaking any bones until the DVDs were completed – I went back on the ice in 2008 for more lessons.

Learning a totally new skill in my sixties was tough. Trying to programme my brain so that my weight was on the right part of the skate and my hands were in one position while my knees were in another seemed impossible. The other challenge was coming to terms with the fact that the surface I was on was very slippery, very hard and totally unforgiving if I fell. It was the most mentally challenging thing I have done in years – but I love it and I wouldn't be driving an hour each way to the nearest rink whenever I can squeeze half a day out of my busy life if I didn't!

I'm not very good, but my coach, Karen Goodwin, fortunately has the patience of Job. With work commitments stretching my diary, I don't skate as often as I would like but Karen has helped me reach a level where I can at least go forwards and backwards reasonably comfortably. I was asked to audition for *Dancing on Ice* twice more but sadly I didn't make the final selection. I realise that I'm probably too old now to be considered – it's such a dangerous and physically demanding sport – but the standard of the skating has now reached such a high level that there's no doubt if I were to be included, it would be very, very tough.

One of the biggest problems with retirement – and why I will never retire completely – is that the spark of being very busy and meeting deadlines and pressures is brilliant for keeping you sharp and mentally fit. I still get a buzz when there's a new project or idea to work on. I thrive on it. Whether it's working in our business, organising charity events or public speaking – they all stretch me and challenge me and when they work they are immensely rewarding mentally.

Don't misunderstand me. I *love* my holidays and we probably have more holidays now than we've ever had, but after a couple of weeks I get bored – my brain gets bored – and I have to start writing something or plan an event, even if it's only in my head. I would go nuts if I wasn't busy. Fortunately, my husband, Mike, understands this and has accepted that I will always be active and on the go. Let's hope that's why he loved me in the first place!

I asked Raj about the evidence that having a positive attitude can help us to live longer:

Raj explained that there has been quite a lot of research on this subject and the idea that optimists live longer than pessimists. There may be all sorts of reasons for that and one of them could be something to do with the behaviours you perform as a result of being an optimist. For example, if you're an optimist you might believe that you would lose weight if you went on a diet plan. A pessimist would think there's no point. Optimists believe there are gains to be had by trying to be healthier and this approach to life is the reason why they live longer.

Another interesting point is optimists are nicer to be around and so they tend to have a wider social circle, which is maybe why they live for longer. They have a reason to live, a circle of support, with other people around them. According to Raj, that's why it's very important to be thinking about the idea that as we get older our lives are getting better and better and don't take a negative view of old age.

My mother-in-law Jeanne lives with us. Jeanne is in her 90th year and the most positive person I know. She's as bright as a button, needs no aid to her hearing or walking, and her eyesight is as good as mine. She is highly motivated, makes all her own Christmas and birthday cards and does any sewing jobs that we need doing – and loves doing them.

Last year we were given a pile of cosmetics by the various beauty house concessions in Boots in Leicester as prizes for our tombola for a large, charity fundraising concert called Music in the Meadow, which we hold in our grounds each August bank holiday. I asked Jeanne if she would make little cellophane parcels of the cosmetics and tie each one with ribbon. She had a couple of weeks to complete the job, but Jeanne was on to it immediately. In two days she had completed 35 exquisitely presented packages, all trimmed with curly ribbon and designed so they would stand up unaided on the tombola stall.

I was extremely grateful for Jeanne's efforts and hard work. And Jeanne got a new lease of life. Suddenly she felt needed and useful again – a lesson I took on board and so I don't feel guilty when I ask her to do jobs for us. Soon I was finding cushions from around the house that our late German Shepherd, Max, had split open, as she loved pulling off the tags from zips! Jeanne sewed up each of the cushions and told me how her fingers 'were really quite stiff now –

and aching'. I apologised for giving her such strong fabric to sew, but instead of moaning she said, 'Oh no, I must use my hands more so they get stronger.' What a fantastic attitude.

On telling this story to Raj he explained that as we get older a lot of people take the view that they're not needed because they think other people can do things better. Needing to be needed is really important and that relates to one's confidence about oneself, which leads on to taking physical exercise. Exercise gives you more confidence. The less exercise you do, the less confident you feel about your ability to do stuff and the more worried you are about falling over. He went on to explain that there is something called 'space phobia', which sounds a strange idea, but older people tend to develop it. They get the idea that in a space they are going to fall over. The more active they have been in the past, the less likely they are to form that phobia of falling over. So that's another reason why we should be more interested in taking up exercise as we get older rather than doing less.

As if we didn't need any more convincing that exercise has a really important role to play in the anti-ageing process, we should remember that as we get older our metabolic rate slows down quite dramatically. If we want to eat a reasonable amount of food and still stay trim, the answer is to increase our level of activity and exercise. It doesn't have to be anything exhausting. I'm certainly not suggesting that you take up jogging or running – in fact I wouldn't recommend that at all – but a good long walk every day could be life-changing. Working out to a fitness DVD is perfect and playing golf, tennis, badminton, gardening, swimming, cycling are all brilliant. Not only will you be healthier, but you will also enjoy the many benefits of being able to move about easily without the handicap of being overweight. There has never been a better case for doing extra exercising to stay young. Just do it!

Visit www.rosemaryconley.tv to see my interview with Raj Persaud on the psychology of ageing.

GOLDEN RULES FOR A YOUTHFUL MIND
- Exercise more.
- Develop a positive attitude.
- Learn new skills.
- Mix with positive people.
- Take up a new sport.

12
Hormone replacement therapy (HRT)

Hormone replacement therapy is a miracle medication, as any woman who has experienced the discomfort of hot flushes, night sweats, anxiety attacks, lack of confidence, exhaustion and low moods as they go through the 'change' can testify. Going through the menopause can be a miserable experience.

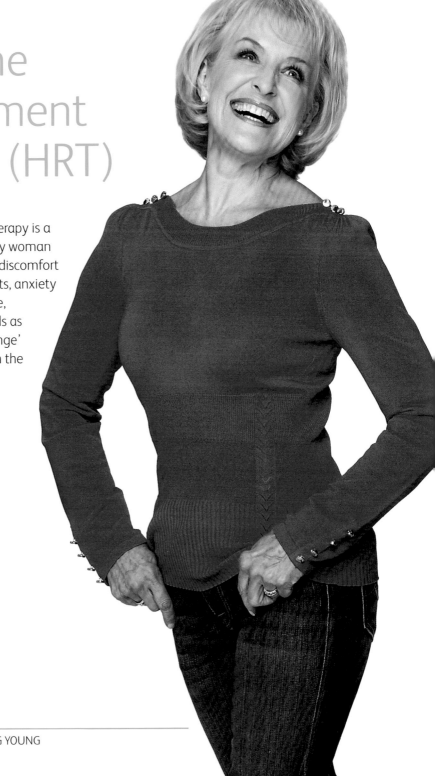

I had a hysterectomy when I was 33 but I still had my ovaries. Having a hysterectomy was brilliant. No more inconvenience or discomfort of periods and it transformed how I felt for 20 years. If your GP or specialist recommends that you have a hysterectomy, then go ahead and don't be frightened. Once you are over the operation you'll be amazed how much better you feel, though it does take a while to get back to full fitness. And, by the way, having a hysterectomy didn't make me age prematurely nor did it make me fat – two of the myths associated with the operation!

However, when I reached my early 50s I suddenly found myself feeling lifeless, 'old', unmotivated, tired – all the things I had never felt before. I went to the doctor to find out what was wrong. A blood test revealed that I was 'perimenopausal', which means I was beginning to go through the menopause.

I'd always thought I wouldn't go on HRT. I was fit and healthy and felt I wouldn't need it but my doctor had other ideas. He suggested I try an oestrogen-only HRT patch. As I had no womb I didn't need the dual HRT, which would have included progesterone.

So I applied my patch to my abdomen and waited to see what happened. Within a couple of weeks I felt like a new woman. The effect was incredible and I've never looked back. I've been on HRT for 12 years now and I want to stay on it for life. It really is a miracle drug and one that has transformed my life.

Whenever I go for a medical, the consulting doctor asks me how long I've been on HRT and when I tell them, they say, 'Normally we recommend that people should only stay on it for a few years,' and then explain the tiny risk of breast cancer – because, I'm told, they are requested to do so. I explain that I want to stay on it for life and that because I'm at a healthy weight, exercise regularly and don't smoke and have no family history of breast cancer, my chances of getting breast cancer are very small anyway. They always agree and the female doctor I saw last time said, 'I'm staying on it too! I agree with you.'

In preparing to write this chapter I consulted with Dr Hilary Jones, as I was interested to know what he thought and was delighted to find that he agreed with my opinion on the subject. The following information and comments are based on Dr Hilary's experience as a GP and mine as a user.

Types of HRT

HRT is available in tablet and patch formats. Most of them are synthetic and they directly mimic the human hormones oestrogen and progesterone. The benefit of patches is that the hormones are absorbed more easily into the body so only a lower dose is necessary, compared with tablets, which have to pass through the body and be processed by the liver before releasing the hormones, and therefore require a higher dose to achieve the same effect.

Some women are given HRT in tablet form and find that it doesn't suit them. They then come off it, thinking that HRT isn't right for them. But there are so many different brands of HRT, and if they had tried a different one, it could have had a transforming effect on their body and their lives. A staggering 60 per cent of women who go on HRT come off it within three months, which, in my opinion, is a real shame. They have abandoned it just because they haven't found the one that's right for them. So if you've had a bad experience, it may be worth having a chat with your GP to see if you could try an alternative.

Dr Hilary explained to me that witnessing the benefits enjoyed by women who take HRT is one of the most rewarding experiences for a GP.

If you still have your womb and your ovaries and you're going through the menopause, you will be given combined HRT, which contains both oestrogen and progesterone. If you were given oestrogen-only HRT, it could lead to a build up in the lining of the womb, which should be avoided. If you've had a hysterectomy, you will be given oestrogen-only HRT.

What are the risks – and the benefits?

A few years ago there was a report indicating that HRT greatly increased your chances of getting breast cancer. The media jumped on it and women in their thousands abandoned their HRT. A couple of years later, the scare was reversed and it was proven that the health benefits from HRT outweighed the very small increased risk of breast cancer. This received significantly less publicity and, unfortunately in my view, many women didn't go back to their GP for more treatment. Dr Hilary explained that the scare was out of proportion to the risks and that it's much easier to scare people than it is to reassure them. Let's hope this book will help to reassure women to try again so that they can get their life back.

I believe the benefits from HRT are absolutely amazing. Here are just a few: as mentioned earlier, HRT protects against the brittle bone disease osteoporosis – and that is key; it preserves our collagen levels, which in turn helps prevent stress incontinence; it can help prevent memory loss; it can reduce levels of anxiety; and it can significantly reduce hot flushes and night sweats. Psychologically, we will feel more confident, our libido will increase, our sexual function will be maintained, our skin won't become so dry so we'll have fewer wrinkles, our hair density will be retained for longer and it will feel stronger and be less brittle.

Earlier I mentioned that the reason everything begins to droop and sag as we women get older is because our oestrogen levels fall, which directly affects our levels of collagen. HRT obviously will boost our oestrogen levels, not only in our skin, breasts and body but also in the brain. Yes, it's great to have firm breasts and better skin, but if we boost the oestrogen in the brain, our minds can be sharper, too, and we'll be less forgetful, brighter and more able to concentrate. And that gives us the all-important 'X factor': confidence. HRT truly is life-changing.

So, *is* there an increased risk of breast cancer? First of all the risk is tiny – 0.1 per cent. One in nine of us will get breast cancer anyway, so the tiny increased risk is on top of an already small risk. That risk can be offset if we are screened regularly and get into the habit of practising breast self-examination to look for any changes. If there are, have them checked out immediately.

The only women for whom HRT is not recommended are those who have a history of breast cancer in the family and it wouldn't be offered to them anyway as their GP would no doubt be aware of their family history.

Dr Hilary agrees that, provided there is no personal or family history of breast cancer, no predisposition to blood clots and no pre-existing medical condition that might be affected by HRT, then there is no reason why we shouldn't be on HRT for life. I know I certainly will.

HRT has transformed my life and I wouldn't be able to lead the active, busy life that I do without it. The brand I use is Estraderm 100 and I change my patch twice a week. And yes, it really is magical.

GOLDEN RULES FOR HRT
- Check with your GP if HRT could be an option for you.
- If you've had an unsatisfactory first attempt with HRT, ask if you could try again.
- Accept any breast screening/mammograms that are offered to you.
- Self-examine your breasts regularly.
- If you still have a womb, accept cervical screening whenever it is offered.

For more information, log on to www.rosemaryconley.tv to see Dr Hilary Jones and me discussing HRT.

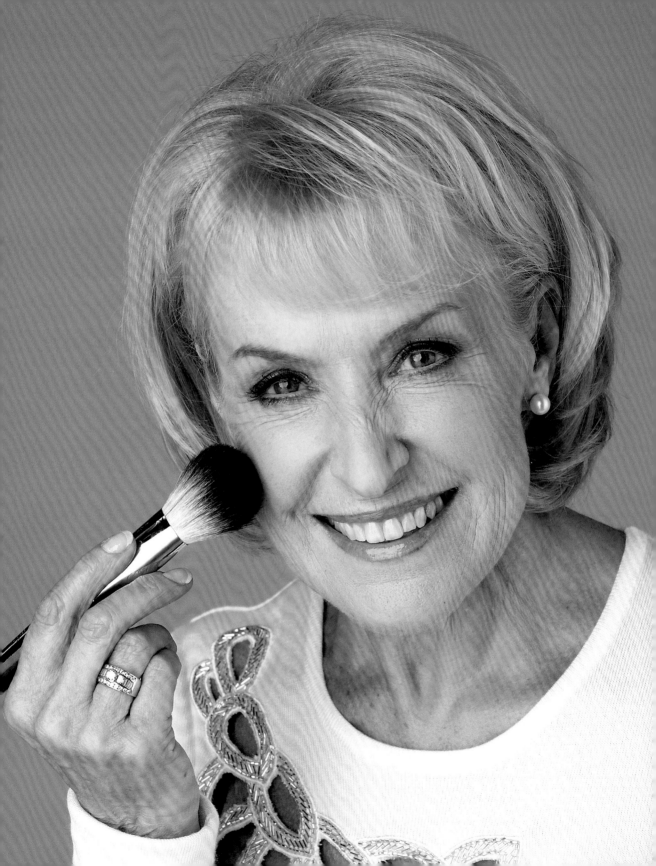

13
Makeup: What to use and how to use it

It was in the early 1980s that I made my first television appearance. *Central Tonight* was a news programme for the Midlands that went out around 6 p.m. I'd been invited to discuss a *Which?* report that had just been published on the virtues of butter compared with margarine. I don't remember very much about the interview but I *do* remember how the makeup artist transformed my looks with her skill and expertise. I wanted her to come and live at our house!

Since that very nervous first experience of the small screen I've had the pleasure of appearing on television many times and have had thousands of photographs taken of me – after I have been professionally made up. Consequently, I've learned a massive amount from these artists about how to apply cosmetics, how to make the most of my face by enhancing the good bits and minimising the not-so-good bits.

Over the years I have tried lots of different cosmetics. Some were recommended to me by makeup artists; others I discovered myself. But one thing is for sure – everything I recommend on these pages are items I have personally tried and love.

Preparing the face

Just as an artist prepares their canvas before creating their next masterpiece, so we need to prepare our face with a moisturiser that suits our skin type. A moisturiser does two jobs. First, it protects our skin from the elements, creating a barrier between our skin and the makeup. Secondly, it adds a layer of moisture to our skin to enable cosmetics to be applied evenly. If we don't use a moisturiser, our foundation cream will look uneven and blotchy as the drier areas of skin will absorb a greater amount. Not using a moisturiser is potentially asking for trouble.

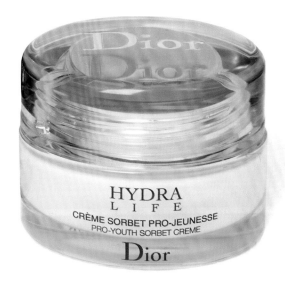

There are products that combine a moisturiser and a tinted foundation and these can work if you don't have a dry skin. Trial and error is the only way to establish whether these suit you. Personally, I don't like them but that's because I have dry skin.

I use Dior Hydra Life Pro-youth Comfort Cream. I like its freshness and light feel and yet it's really effective in moisturising my skin ready for my foundation cream.

Magnifying mirror

Unless you have good eyesight that allows you to see easily close-up, you'll need a magnifying mirror to use when applying your makeup. They come in a variety of strengths from double magnification to 10x strength! These are quite frightening and can make us look 10 years older – remember, though, that's not how the world sees us. A magnifying mirror does, however, allow us to do a professional job in applying our makeup. There's nothing worse than not being able to see where you are applying your eyeshadow or eyeliner.

Also remember that when you look in the mirror first thing in the morning, you will look at your worst. That image is not what the world will see by the time you have given your face a chance to 'wake up'. It takes a few hours, particularly as we get older, for our face to regulate itself. First thing in the morning our eyes are puffy, skin looks dull and our eyes look tired. This will pass. Just give it time.

My tip here is to buy the best magnifying mirror you can afford. The better the quality of the mirror, the more accurate the image. Poor-quality mirrors can distort our features and make us look pretty grim.

Why do we need a magnifying mirror? To be able to spot the odd whisker peeping its unattractive presence into sight, the odd stray nose hair, hair growing out of a mole and the dreaded moustache! Getting older is so attractive isn't it?

And there's nothing worse than someone saying to you, 'Oh, you have an eyelash on your face, let me remove it,' only to find it's attached to your cheek!

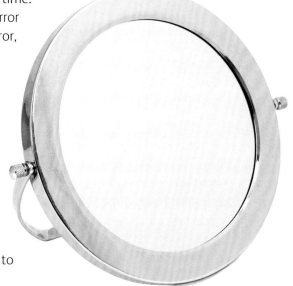

Travel magnifying mirror.

Brushes or sponges?

I've never been a fan of sponges because they soak up too much foundation cream, which means a lot gets wasted. I prefer to use brushes to apply all my makeup as I find it's easier, you

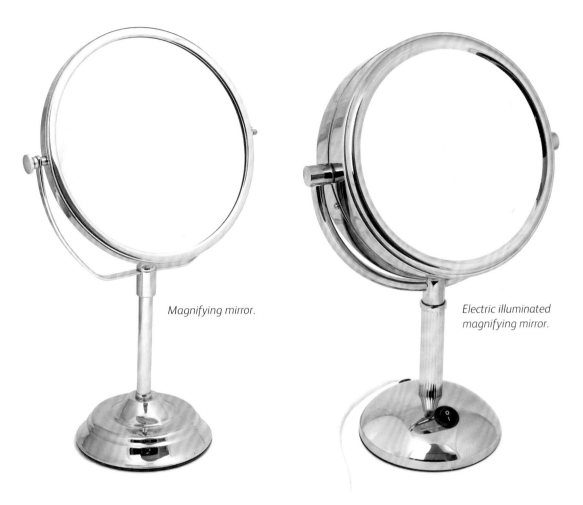

Magnifying mirror.

Electric illuminated magnifying mirror.

only use the amount of product you need and the end result is more flattering. By using the right brush for the various jobs – foundation, eyeshadow, powder, blusher – you can achieve a much more professional look and finish.

Brushes can be easily cleaned in soapy water but as you are using them only on yourself, they don't need cleaning every day. You can buy a brush-cleaner, which is a quick-drying dissolvent that cleans the brushes swiftly and hygienically, but this tends to be used more by makeup artists who are reusing their brushes on another client almost immediately.

Brushes vary enormously in quality and there are many to choose from. After much searching, I've selected what I consider to be the best-quality brushes for the job and I've described their different uses below. Because good brushes are expensive, I decided to put together a set that's now available to buy through my website. These are the ones that I use all the time and could not manage without. You may choose to buy your brushes on the high street but hopefully this guide will help to prevent some expensive mistakes.

1 Dual-length foundation brush: Made up of bristles of two different lengths, this brush is brilliant for applying foundation cream. Just gently apply the cream to your face with small circular movements, almost as if you were massaging your face with the brush. Remember to go right up to the hairline, past your jawline and blend into your neckline. This brush gives a very natural covering all over the face and eyes and goes into all the crevices and corners very effectively.

2 Powder brush: Whether you are using loose powder or a compact, always apply your powder with a brush and not a powder puff or sponge. Pat the powder on rather than drag it. By using a brush you'll achieve a lighter covering but one that will 'set' your foundation and keep it looking good all day. Avoid the temptation to apply too much as you will run the risk of your makeup 'cracking' and that's not a good look.

3 Eye highlighter brush: This brush is used to apply a cream or light-coloured eyeshadow to your eyelids and up to your eyebrows. It needs to be soft to use on the thin skin on the eyelid, but strong enough to apply the light eyeshadow smoothly.

4 and 5 Eye socket brushes: These brilliant little brushes make eyeshadow application really easy. Their pointed ends mean they are very effective for applying your chosen eyeshadow to your eye socket, which makes your eyes look bigger and wider. I also use this style of brush to apply a triangle of darker shadow to the outside corners of my eyes. This adds depth and width to the eyes.

6 Blusher brush: It's really important to get this brush right. If you buy one that's too dense, you're likely to apply too much blusher in a small area. A soft and flexible brush will effectively add a little 'blush' to your cheekbones without overdoing it. Aim for the 'apples' of your cheeks when you smile.

7 Eyebrow brush/eyelash comb: This brush is useful for brushing your eyebrows into shape, and the comb helps to separate eyelashes that may become stuck together with mascara.

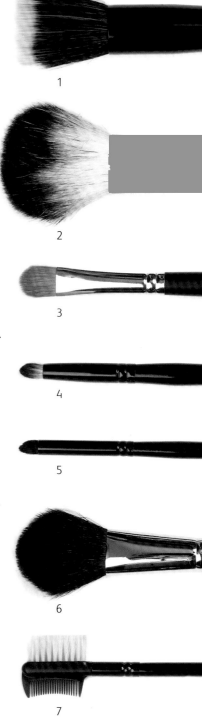

Makeup and how to apply it

After moisturising, apply your makeup in the following order:

- Concealer (apply to total eyelid area and to dark circles under eyes)
- Foundation cream
- Powder
- Highlight eyeshadow
- Eyeshadow (eye socket)
- Eyeshadow (outer corner of eyelid)
- Eyeliner (if using)
- Mascara
- Lip liner (if using)
- Lipstick/lip gloss
- Blusher

What cosmetics do I need?

Concealer: Using a cosmetic concealer helps to hide the dark circles we may find under our eyes. As we age, the skin under our eyes can become puffy and lined and the colour of the skin under our eyes and on our eyelids can become darker. The texture of the skin in this area is also very thin and delicate.

I use a concealer by Dior, called Diorskin Nude Natural Glow Hydrating Makeup, which I apply with the tips of my third fingers under my eyes and also across my eyelids and up to my eyebrows. This has the effect of lightening the darker skin in this area but it also helps my eye makeup to stay in place once applied. I smooth the light-coloured cream under my eyes to include the dark semi-circles. I apply this before my foundation cream.

If I feel it's necessary, I may add a little more concealer over the 'dark semi-circles' under my eyes once I've applied my foundation, depending on how dark the circles are, or how big the bags might be on any one day! I apply it with a very thin artist's brush for best effect or I use Healthspan Nurture's Illuminating Touch Treatment Concealer click pen, which is very easy to apply. You can also use concealer on either side of your nostrils and in the crease

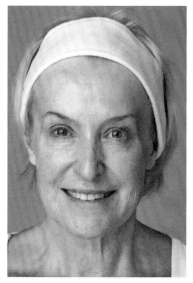

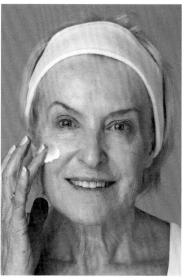

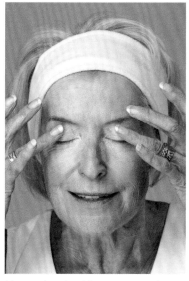

This is my face without any makeup. Note the pinkiness underneath and above the eyes caused by the skin thinning with age.

Apply your moisturiser before your makeup.

Using the third finger on each hand, apply a liquid concealer to the eyelids up to the eyebrows and underneath the eyes.

between your cheeks and nose to soften the appearance of lines.

Of course, the most famous concealer on the market is Touche Éclat by Yves Saint Laurent. Personally I prefer the Dior and Healthspan Nurture products because I think they cover the skin better. But, for a quick touch-up under the eye once you've applied your makeup, Touche Éclat is good, and many a makeup artist swears by it. However, I always keep the Healthspan pen in my handbag for emergency touching-up.

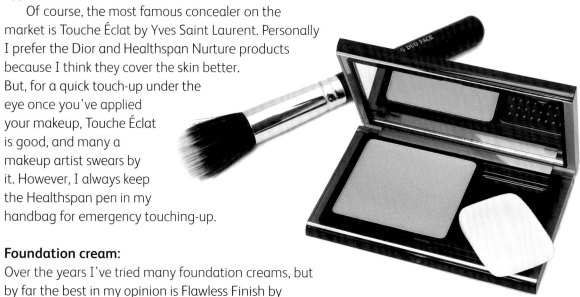

Foundation cream:

Over the years I've tried many foundation creams, but by far the best in my opinion is Flawless Finish by

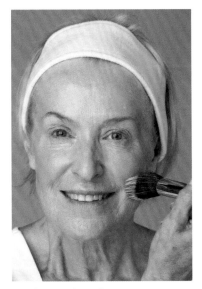

Apply your foundation cream in circular movements across the entire face with a dual-length brush. The circular movement of the brush ensures total coverage of any wrinkles to give an even finish.

Elizabeth Arden. This is a cream foundation packed in a compact with a sponge for application. As mentioned earlier, I'm not a fan of sponges because they 'soak up' too much foundation, which I feel is wasteful, so I apply Flawless Finish with the dual-length foundation brush. It goes on like a dream and ever since I mentioned this product in my 'Rosemary Recommends' column in my *Diet & Fitness* magazine, all the girls in the magazine office have started using it and swear by it. It's a total hit all round.

Flawless Finish comes in several colours, so ask the Elizabeth Arden consultant on the beauty counter to advise you on what's best for you.

Powder: Loose or compact? This is down to personal choice. For convenience I think a compact is great because it's less messy and easier to apply. I love Lucidity by Estée Lauder, which is translucent, so it doesn't add colour, and it's reflective, which gives a lovely finish without being heavy. Whichever powder you choose, try to select a shade that will not 'add' colour to your foundation, otherwise the finish will be too heavy. Go for one that's translucent or paler than your foundation.

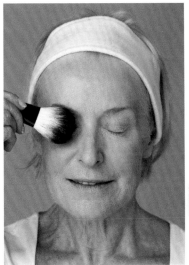

Apply powder lightly, using a patting action, across the entire face with a large powder brush.

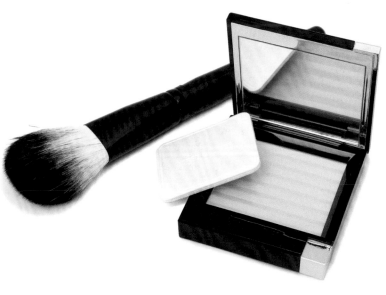

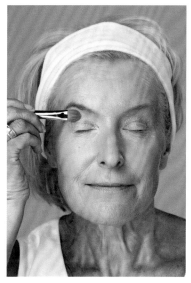
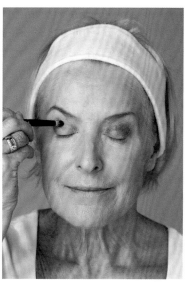
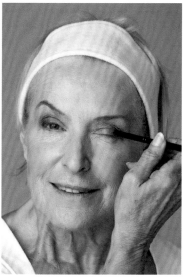

Apply cream or beige highlighter eyeshadow across the whole eye socket up to the eyebrow.

Apply light brown or light grey eyeshadow to the socket line and outer corner of the eyelid.

Apply a darker shade of brown or grey to the outer corner in a triangular shape. Blend the edges as necessary.

Highlight eyeshadow: If there's one area where you can economise on cost, I suggest it's with eyeshadow. I've used great products in the Boots' No7 range and also from L'Oréal. As we get older it's best to avoid shades with sparkle as these tend to show the creases more and can look unflattering. Select colours that are right for you and ask a beauty consultant to help you make the right choice. I tend to go for a cream highlighter shadow rather than white and I avoid pinks as they make me look as if I've been crying!

Coloured eyeshadows: After applying the light shade of base shadow all over my eyelids and up to my eyebrows, I apply a curve of mid brown for the eye socket. I take care not to let it go too far down at the outer corner, as it would bring the look of the eye downwards. For the outer corner triangle I use a dark brown. This gives width and depth to the eye. The colours used here should be subtle, so avoid bright colours completely. Greys – lighter and darker – are great on mature skin, as are browns and beiges. Ask a beauty consultant for guidance.

Eyeliner: Eyeliner is also a matter of personal choice. You need to be able to apply it correctly – and that can be tricky – and it needs to be reasonably subtle. Eyeliner is supposed to add definition to your eyes and make your eyelashes look thicker. Applied well, it can make your eyes look amazing. Applied badly, it can make you look hard and tarty. It comes in liquid form, or as a kohl pencil. I prefer the liquid as I find the kohl pencil too thick and too hard on the delicate skin

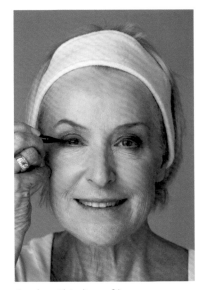

Apply a thin line of brown or grey eyeliner as close to the lashes as possible. Do not go into the inner corner of the eye as this will look too heavy. Use a cotton bud to clear up any smudges.

of the eyelid. I try to go for brown liquid eyeliner, which is subtler on my fair skin and it goes with my beige/brown eyeshadows. If you wear grey eyeshadow, you could try charcoal or gunmetal shades of eyeliner. If you insist on wearing black, don't overdo it or it will add years to you.

Finding the right liquid eyeliner is not easy, but I've found Dior to be the best. To apply it, paint as thin a line as possible, above and close to the upper lashes, starting close to the inner corner, but not quite there, and moving outwards towards the very end of the eyelid. For the undereye area, which needs less liner, take a line from just over halfway along (about a third of the way in from the corner) and paint a line out to the corner to meet the upper line. Keep the line as close as you possibly can to the eyelashes and carefully remove any surplus with a cotton wool bud. With eyeliner, practice definitely makes perfect, and remember that less is more.

Mascara: Mascara is a must to finish off your eye makeup. Even if you don't wear eyeshadow, please wear some mascara – and take your time in applying it. It's really important to apply mascara in the same direction that your eyelashes grow. Again, I prefer brown or brown/black colours for myself,

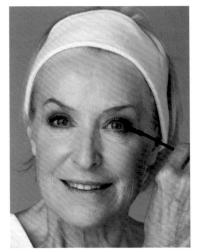

Apply mascara (brown or black, depending on your colouring). Apply to the upper and lower lashes but ensure that the upper lashes are brushed in an outwards direction at the outer corners.

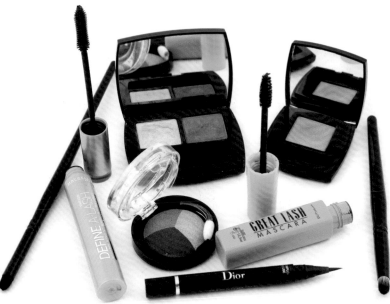

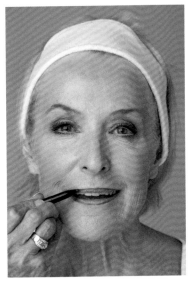

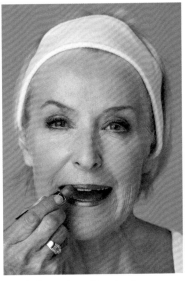

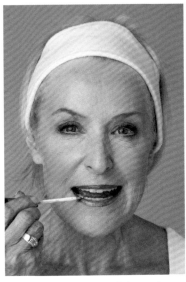

Apply lip liner pencil to give definition to the line of your lips.

Apply lipstick within the lines drawn by the lip liner.

Add lip gloss on top if desired.

but I do sometimes wear black and feel it looks all right. Having experimented with so many different mascaras my favourites are Define-A-Lash and Great Lash, both from Maybelline, though L'Oréal makes some great ones too.

Lip liner: This is an extremely important item in my view. As we get older the contour of our lips becomes less clear and some vertical lines may start to appear, into which our lipstick can bleed. You want to avoid this like the plague. A lip liner acts as a barrier to keep the lipstick colour inside the lip area and it also adds definition to the shape of your lips. I'm not for a moment suggesting that you start applying brown lip liner, as was fashionable in the 1990s, but I am recommending a subtle pink or pale red liner to tone with your lipstick. You really shouldn't be able to see the join. If you

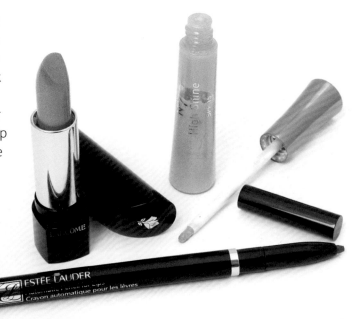

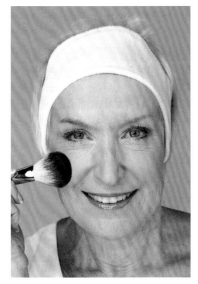

Apply powder blusher to your blusher brush and tap off any excess. Smile and apply to the 'apples' of the cheeks. Apply only a little at a time and add more if necessary.

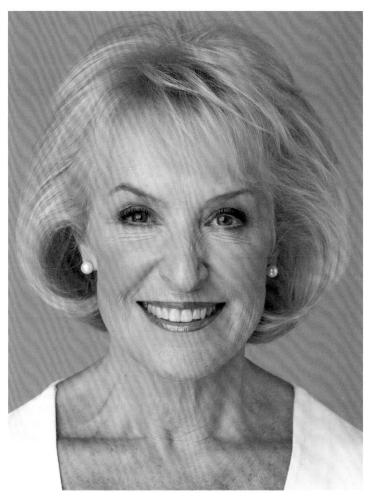

All finished and feeling more like me!

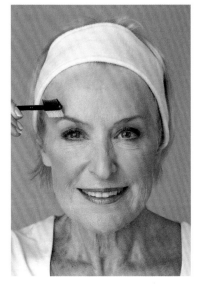

And finally ... brush the eyebrows into shape with an eyebrow brush.

want to wear only lip gloss, you can buy an invisible lip liner that will stop the gloss bleeding and give a controlled 'edge' to your lips.

Lipstick: These days any colour goes and you can see women wearing any shade from dark purple to pale nude. It's down to what you like and trial and error. I don't think pillar-box red looks good on older women or that we should wear anything that's too loud or bold. In my view a good colour for mature skin is a pastel shade so that the makeup looks finished but not brazen.

Lip gloss: You may not wish to wear lip gloss, but it adds shine and gives a lovely finish to your makeup. You can buy coloured ones, which can be worn on their own, or clear ones to add gloss to your lipstick. I use one and it helps to stop me 'eating' my lipstick, which is an annoying habit of mine! Find a gloss you like but don't be surprised if you find it tastes of fruit! Many do, but personally I'm not keen. If I wanted a strawberry taste I'd buy fresh ones. Lancôme does a range that isn't fruity.

Blusher: Blusher is applied last, as the colour from the lipstick helps us to balance how much blusher we need. Use a brush and smile as you apply the blusher to the apples of your cheeks. Use just a little first, then add more if necessary. Once the blusher powder is on the brush, give it a tap to let the excess drop away before application. You don't want to apply too much as, once applied, it's really difficult to tone down.

When you've finished, check over your entire face to see that you haven't left any brush bristles or globules of mascara.

Applying makeup takes practice and confidence. The more you practise, the more confident you will become. One thing is for sure, we *all* look better when we wear makeup no matter what our age. My lovely mother-in-law, Jeanne, always applies hers first thing in the morning without fail – and I'll be doing the same if I reach the wonderful age of 89 too!

GOLDEN RULES FOR APPLYING MAKEUP
- Always apply makeup to a clean and moisturised face.
- Use good-quality brushes for a smooth accurate application of cosmetics.
- Apply your makeup in the correct order.
- Check close-up, in a magnifying mirror, for even application.

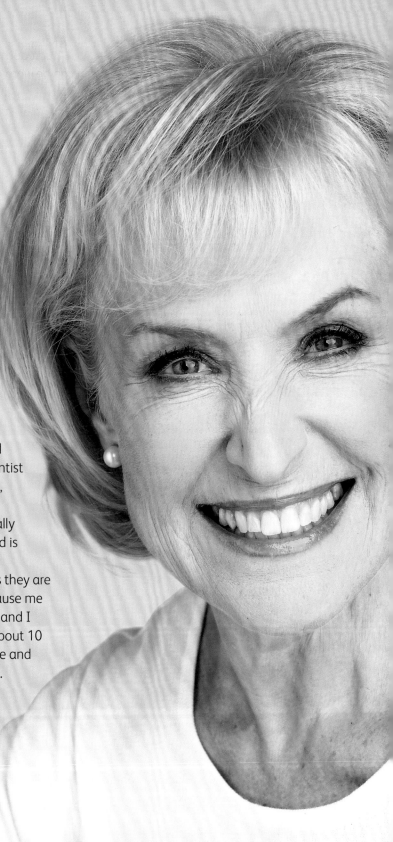

14
Teeth

Our teeth are vitally important to our appearance and a crucial part of keeping us looking youthful. As well as the eyes, the mouth is the focal point of the face as it's what others look at when they are talking to us. Looking at someone's mouth as they speak helps us to hear more easily, and the expression of the mouth helps us to understand the manner and attitude of the person speaking. Our teeth are a key feature and we need to spend time and energy looking after them.

A good diet will help us to have good teeth, as will regular check-ups at the dentist every six months and, while you're there, make an appointment with the dental hygienist. Getting your teeth professionally polished and having any plaque removed is truly a good investment.

I've been fortunate with my teeth as they are naturally quite white and straight and cause me very little trouble. I have very few fillings and I have all my teeth bar one, which I lost about 10 years ago. The gap that it left isn't visible and I manage to eat perfectly well without it.

I look after my teeth by using dental floss and brush them with a medium soft toothbrush morning and night. I use a toothpaste for sensitive teeth as I just have one tooth that is sensitive to hot and cold temperatures. My hygienist tells me that sensitive toothpaste works brilliantly for some people and just doesn't work for others, so it's a question of giving it a try. Colgate Sensitive works for me.

In particular, as we get older we need to look after our gums, and using a brush that is too hard, and in an up-and-down movement, can cause the gums to recede. Over time this means that the part of the tooth normally living inside our gums can become exposed and eventually your tooth could become loose and fall out. To avoid this, use a soft to medium bristle strength and operate your brush in a circular movement over the teeth and gums. It cleans them better and causes significantly less damage.

Electric toothbrushes are great if you like them. There's no doubt they do a good job but, again, it's a matter of personal preference.

A popular cosmetic dental treatment for celebrities is having very bright white veneers fitted to their teeth. A top layer of the natural teeth is removed and veneers are applied over the top. Personally, I think they are too obvious and can look artificial. But if you have very discoloured teeth, and no simple whitening solution can be found, maybe splashing out on veneers would prove a good investment as it can boost your confidence big-time.

'Whitening' toothpastes will certainly help to brighten and lighten your teeth but there's nothing better for your teeth than regular brushing, flossing and visits to the dentist and hygienist and, of course, a healthy diet.

If you have a very visible gap in your teeth when you smile, consider having it corrected. I know dental surgery is expensive, but investing in your smile is definitely worth doing if you can afford it. Perhaps you've learned to live with that missing front tooth and feel it's too late to do anything about it. It isn't. You'll feel such a surge of confidence if you have it sorted out as it will transform your smile and change the way you present yourself in future. And, remember, we want to enjoy to the full every single day that we are alive.

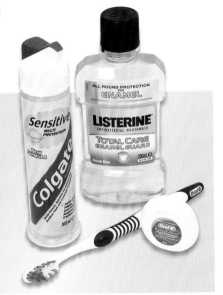

GOLDEN RULES FOR TEETH

- Brush your teeth at least every morning and evening.
- Use a soft or medium strength toothbrush.
- Brush with circular movements.
- Use dental floss between your teeth every day.
- Visit the dentist and dental hygienist every six months.

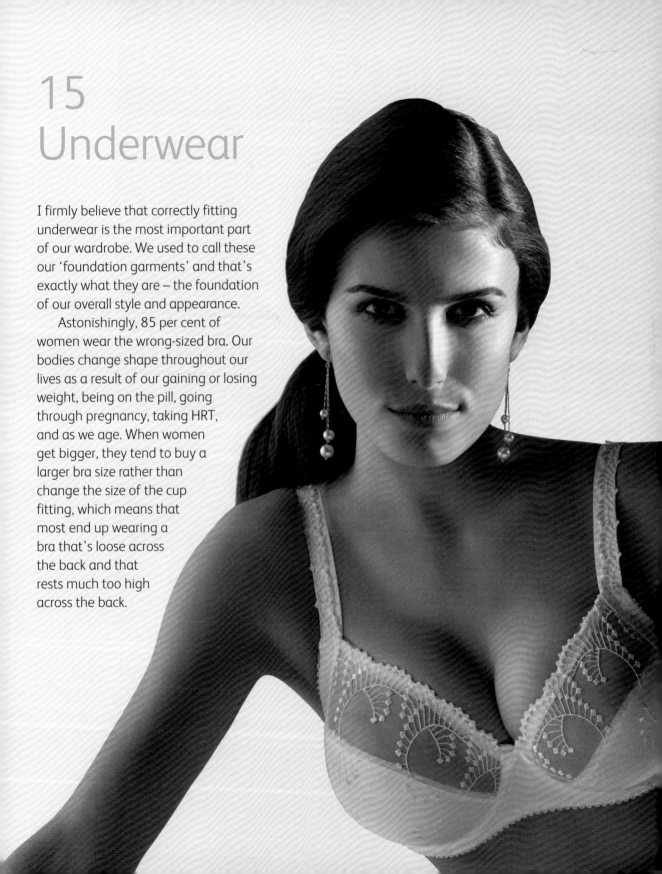

15
Underwear

I firmly believe that correctly fitting underwear is the most important part of our wardrobe. We used to call these our 'foundation garments' and that's exactly what they are – the foundation of our overall style and appearance.

Astonishingly, 85 per cent of women wear the wrong-sized bra. Our bodies change shape throughout our lives as a result of our gaining or losing weight, being on the pill, going through pregnancy, taking HRT, and as we age. When women get bigger, they tend to buy a larger bra size rather than change the size of the cup fitting, which means that most end up wearing a bra that's loose across the back and that rests much too high across the back.

You can quickly spot someone who's wearing the wrong-sized bra by just looking at the position of the back strap. If it's not level with the lower front of the bra, the bra's too big. If you see someone whose bust is 'overflowing' out of the top of their bra cup, then their cup size is too small. Yet when you get it right, the effect is magical.

As we get older our breasts change shape. They often become bigger and they tend to drop from where they were 30 years ago. Wearing a correctly fitting bra that holds your bust in place and lifts and shapes the breasts is vital and yet few women take the time and trouble to be properly fitted and to try different styles to find the right one for them and their unique bosom.

Ever since I was introduced to Rigby and Peller, Corsetieres to the Queen, in London my figure has been transformed. I used to think I was a 34B cup – a size I wore for years – and then, after a professional fitting with Rigby and Peller, I went to 32C. Five years later, I had a refitting and found that I was a 32DD. Having a bigger bust is the very best thing that has happened as I've got older!

The specialist fitters at Rigby and Peller are trained to 'know' what size you are just by looking at you in the mirror. It's a bit odd the first time you go for the fitting and realise that you just have to stand in front of the mirror in the cubicle with your top half naked, but you soon realise that these professionals really do know their stuff. When you try on that bra that makes your boobs look pert and youthful, it's a brilliant boost to your confidence.

I know there are fitting services available in some high street stores and you may find they work for you, but if you have a very slender or very large bust, I urge you to try Rigby and Peller. You won't regret it. You'll need to book an appointment for your fitting and be prepared to pay a bit more for your bra because they are exquisitely styled and beautifully made.

According to June Kenton, the founder of Rigby and Peller, if you were to buy three or four bras a year that fitted you perfectly, you'd probably spend less than if you bought a selection from the high street that didn't fit you so well. I have to agree with her. The bras I've bought from Rigby and Peller have lasted me years longer than high-street ones.

When it comes to pants, how big or how brief you choose them to be is down to you, but I would make two suggestions. Firstly, I always buy the next size up because tight knickers are very uncomfortable, they dig into your flesh and cause bulges under your clothes. Secondly, always choose a style that will not show through your clothes. There's nothing less attractive than seeing a woman in trousers exhibiting the full contour of their pants – it looks awful!

There are plenty of styles available now that are described as NVP – no visible panty-line. Find a style that suits your shape and that you can wear comfortably. I always wear a thong style, which felt a bit strange initially, but now I can't even feel I'm wearing it and it never shows, no matter what I am wearing.

Ever since Trinny and Susannah and Nicky Hambleton-Jones appeared on our television screens, educating us on how to dress to maximise our best features and minimise our worst, wearing support underwear has become acceptable and it's very accessible. Marks and Spencer has a vast range of support underwear in different styles and strengths. That unsightly tummy bulge can be harnessed and a big backside smoothed down in a moment with these garments. Busts can be enhanced with 'chicken fillet' bra inserts or gel-filled bras. What we can do to boost our figure now knows no bounds!

One of the great benefits of wearing 'control' wear is that it gives you a wonderfully smooth, seamless line under your clothes. The key here is not to buy too small a size, as this would cause your flesh and fat to 'overflow'. June Kenton says, 'Leave your fat where you've grown it, and control it there, then your clothes will feel comfortable so you can wear the control garment every day if you wish.'

If you don't have a waist because you're apple-shaped, you could treat yourself to a waist-cincher. This is a modern-day corset that uses hooks and eyelets for the fastening and it has the brilliant effect of giving you a waist if you don't normally have one. We use waist-cinchers occasionally for our slimmers' photo shoots where a style of dress calls for some shape around the waist area. Our dieting superstar models are always thrilled with the results when they see the effect on their figures in their photographs.

Finally, a couple of words of advice: firstly, as you get older your skin becomes looser, so if you're wearing a foundation garment, make sure you've 'tucked in' any surplus flesh. This applies to your bra too. It's worth looking in a reverse mirror before you step out to see the world. Also, remember that exercising regularly will dramatically improve your skin tone as well as your body shape, and holding your tummy in all the time is the best 'corset' you could ever have.

GOLDEN RULES FOR CHOOSING UNDERWEAR

- Get yourself professionally measured for a bra.
- If you have a really heavy or particularly small bust, go to Rigby and Peller for a specialist assessment and sizing.
- Make sure that any support garments are the right size for you and not too tight.
- Wear pants that don't show under your clothes.
- Always check in the reverse mirror for flesh overhang!

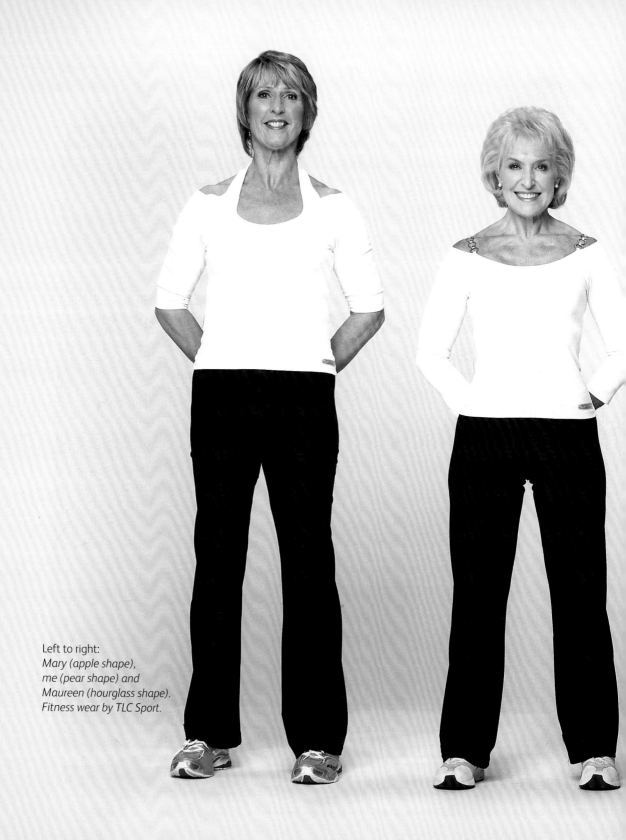

Left to right:
*Mary (apple shape),
me (pear shape) and
Maureen (hourglass shape).
Fitness wear by TLC Sport.*

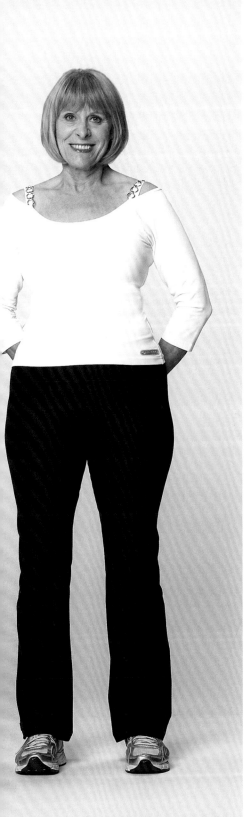

16
Introducing the Stay Young Body Shape Workouts

Your body shape is determined at birth, but as you get older that shape becomes more pronounced as body fat tends to deposit itself more prolifically in those already slightly fatter areas. If you're pear-shaped, your bottom and thighs get bigger; if you're apple-shaped, your tummy gets fatter and your waist thicker; and if you have an hourglass shape, your bust gets larger.

With the help of Mary Morris, my personal exercise consultant and the oracle of all things to do with fitness, I have created a special fitness programme that includes an optimum shape-up programme to suit each body type. Do this programme regularly, and you can have a great figure as you get older and be able to say goodbye to a flat bottom if you're apple-shaped, disproportionate thighs if you're pear-shaped, and a top-heavy bust if you're an hourglass shape.

Know your body shape

To help you decipher your own body shape there's a simple calculation you can do. Using the waist-to-hip ratio test (see over), you can determine for sure which category you fall into if you're unsure. With that information you can go straight to the Stay Young workout that's appropriate for your body shape in Chapters 17 to 19.

Using a tape measure, place it around your waist approximately 2.5cm (1in) above your navel, then jot down your waist measurement. Now place the tape around the widest part of your lower body (check in a mirror to see where this is) and record your hip measurement. Make sure you hold the tape loosely so you can still slide the tape around while standing up straight. Using a calculator, simply divide your waist measurement by your hip measurement.

Result

A measurement of 0.8 or lower means you are a pear shape (or an hourglass if you have a full bust as well as large thighs).

A measurement that is higher than 0.8 means you are an apple shape.

Main Features for Each Body Shape

Pear	Apple	Hourglass
• Larger lower body and smaller upper body	• Bigger on the top half of the body	• Well-proportioned upper and lower body
• Fat stored on bottom, hips and thighs	• Thick waist	• Bigger bust
• Slim waist	• Full bust	• Shoulders and hips a similar width
• Narrow shoulders	• Flattish bottom	• Shapely waist
• Small bust	• Slim hips and thighs	• Curvy figure
• Flattish tummy	• Slim arms and legs	

What is your BMI?

If you are very overweight, it may be more difficult to determine your body shape accurately, so it's important to check your body mass index (BMI) and work towards a healthy weight. BMI is used to establish just how overweight you are and helps you move through the different levels of overweight to reach a healthy goal. To calculate your BMI log on to www.nhs.uk/Tools/Pages/Healthyweightcalculator.aspx or check the charts below to see if your BMI falls into a healthy range.

> BMI less than 18.5 – underweight
> BMI 18.5 to 24.9 – healthy weight
> BMI 25 to 29.9 – overweight
> BMI 30+ – obese

Target height to weight ratio

This handy chart shows the recommended height to weight ratio for your BMI to fall into a healthy range.

HEALTHY HEIGHT/WEIGHT RATIOS

Height without shoes		TARGET BMI 18.5–24.9 Healthy weight range	
4ft 10in	(1.47m)	6st 11lb–8st 7lb	(43.2–54.0kg)
4ft 11in	(1.50m)	7st 1lb–8st 12lb	(45.0–56.3kg)
5ft 0in	(1.52m)	7st 4lb–9st 2lb	(46.2–57.8kg)
5ft 1in	(1.55m)	7st 8lb–9st 7lb	(48.0–60.1kg)
5ft 2in	(1.57m)	7st 11lb–9st 10lb	(49.3–61.6kg)
5ft 3in	(1.60m)	8st 1lb–10st 1lb	(51.2–64kg)
5ft 4in	(1.63m)	8st 5lb–10st 6lb	(53.1–66.4kg)
5ft 5in	(1.65m)	8st 8lb–10st 10lb	(54.5–68.1kg)
5ft 6in	(1.68m)	8st 12lb–11st 2lb	(56.4–70.6kg)
5ft 7in	(1.70m)	9st 2lb–11st 6lb	(57.8–72.3kg)
5ft 8in	(1.73m)	9st 6lb–11st 11lb	(59.9–74.9kg)
5ft 9in	(1.75m)	9st 9lb–12st 1lb	(61.2–76.6kg)
5ft 10in	(1.78m)	10st–12st 7lb	(63.4–79.2kg)
5ft 11in	(1.80m)	10st 3lb–12st 11lb	(64.8–81.0kg)
6ft 0in	(1.83m)	10st 8lb–13st 3lb	(67.0–83.7kg)
6ft 1in	(1.85m)	10st 11lb–13st 7lb	(68.5–85.6kg)
6ft 2in	(1.88m)	11st 2lb–13st 13lb	(70.7–88.4kg)

How the programme works

The body shape toning workouts in the next three chapters are designed to help you shape up and slim down your bigger bits and to strengthen your weaker areas to give your figure a more balanced appearance, so choose the workout that's appropriate for your body shape.

In addition to completing this workout two to three times a week, you should undertake some aerobic fitness activity every day to keep you fit and to burn fat. Combining toning exercises, which use resistance to strengthen the muscles, with some daily aerobic exercise will transform your body shape and your health, helping you to look and feel years younger. For each programme I've recommended which of my fitness DVDs is suitable for your body shape and for each body shape I've also suggested a weekly exercise plan.

Each body shape toning workout in the following chapters has the choice of two toning programmes: one uses light handweights (½–1kg weights or ½ litre water bottles) to make the muscles work harder, and the other uses a resistance band. Using a band causes the muscles to work against greater resistance, which increases the effectiveness of each exercise. If you have a band and can use it comfortably, this is the most effective programme, although alternating between the two toning programmes would be brilliant for maximising the results to your body shape. If you don't own a band, you can obtain one through our website. They are inexpensive and will last you for years.

The fitness programme incorporates three elements – cardiovascular exercise, resistance and toning exercise, and stretching – each of which is really important. It's a progressive programme so that you can develop your strength as you become fitter and more familiar with the exercises. Seeing yourself progressing will keep you motivated and challenged. Here's an explanation of what the programme covers to ensure a complete shape-up.

1 Cardiovascular exercise

To lose weight you will need to do some cardio, or aerobic, exercise to get your heart and lungs working hard, so that your body uses up plenty of calories, burns fat and gets a lot fitter. Aerobic exercise also speeds up your metabolism for hours after your workout, which means you will burn extra calories even when you've stopped exercising. Each body shape workout includes a cardio programme and it doesn't matter whether you choose to get out in the fresh air or get a sweat on in a class or in your local gym. It all counts.

2 Resistance and toning exercise

This part of the programme will help tone you up and sculpt your body to give you a better figure shape and more balanced proportions. Each body shape requires specific toning exercises, using water bottles/handweights or a resistance band to increase their effectiveness. The greater your muscle mass the higher your metabolic rate, so this type of strength training will genuinely help to speed up your metabolism. As your muscles get firmer and denser they will become even more efficient at burning fat when you do your aerobic exercise.

3 Stretching

Whatever your body shape, you will need to complete your workout with a short stretch programme. The choice of stretches depends on the specific exercises you've done in your workout so that you only stretch the muscles you have worked. Each stretch is performed once only and held static for 10 seconds unless otherwise stated. It's at the point when you hold the stretch static that you feel the muscles lengthening and stretching. Stretching increases our flexibility, which is very important as we get a little older, and it also ensures that we release any tension in our muscles so they don't ache as a result of the exercise we've been doing.

Choosing the right level of exercise for you

Each body shape toning workout can be done at two levels – beginners and intermediate. And, remember, you can choose to do the routine that uses handweights or the one that uses a resistance band, to make your workout even more effective. If you prefer, you can do the workout without using equipment.

Beginners

You may want to follow this level if you've not done any formal exercise for a good while or are very overweight. If you do too much too soon, you run a high risk of injury, so please listen to your body. If it starts to hurt, that's a sign to stop, but if it's just a bit uncomfortable, that's normal and it shows you are challenging your muscles, which is good.

Intermediate

This level is for experienced exercisers who want to be challenged. The recommended number of repetitions is only a guide, but useful for those who are not sure about how much is safe and effective. If you have the stamina to work really hard, your capability to burn more calories is greatly enhanced as the calories will keep on burning at a higher rate even after you stop exercising.

How to use this programme

- Identify your body shape, using the waist-to-hip ratio on page 110.
- Write down your start weight and your BMI on the chart on pages 137 (pear), 163 (apple) or 188 (hourglass).
- Follow the plan designed exclusively for your body shape.

- Every month, record your new weight and BMI.
- Some exercises include handweights or a resistance band. You can use water bottles instead of handweights and you can buy the resistance band online at www.rosemaryconley.com. All exercises can be done without equipment if you prefer.

Useful training tips
- Keep some water handy to stay hydrated.
- Always warm up before any exercise programme. With cardio (aerobic) work, start gently and increase the intensity gradually. For resistance/toning exercises, either go for a brisk five-minute walk, swinging the arms, or march on the spot for 3 minutes, circling the shoulders and lifting alternate knees higher after every 20 steps.
- If you're new to exercise, use only ½ litre water bottles for the resistance exercises or no weights.
- To cool down after your aerobic exercise, always reduce the intensity gradually and finish with the post-cardio stretches on pages 138 (pear), 164 (apple) or 189 (hourglass).

17
The Stay Young Pear Shape Workout

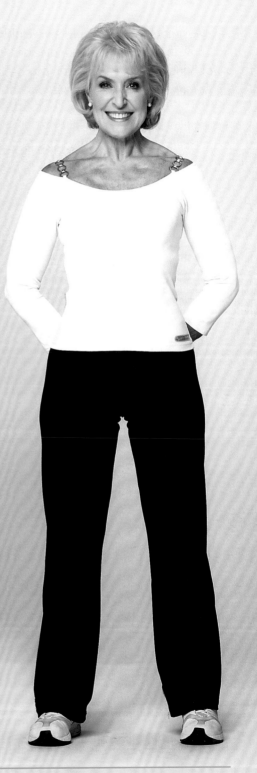

If you're a pear shape, you will store fat around your hips and thighs, which could be said is where nature intended it to be stored. It's all linked to fertility and childbearing. However, the upside is that you'll have a flatter stomach than most other shapes and an enviable waistline, so let's make the most of these good parts.

Because a pear shape's arms and legs carry more fat, compared with other body shapes, you're at greater risk of having 'wobbly bits' in these areas as you get older. There's a lot you can do to help keep your arms and legs toned, but you have to work at it.

It's a good idea to work on your chest and shoulders, too, as making these areas stronger and giving them good muscle definition will help to balance your wider lower half so that you appear slimmer. You can emphasise this balance even more by dressing carefully – more about that in Chapter 21.

The problem for pear shapes is that the fat stored around the hips and thighs is notoriously hard to shift. But, with regular fat-burning aerobic exercise and some concentrated toning moves, combined with a low-fat diet, miracles can happen. Losing weight is the key to getting slimmer legs, but exercise is vital for a lovely shape.

The best exercise for your shape

Even if you're a pear shape and a healthy weight, you may feel your thighs are still a problem. As well as working the hips and thighs, these exercises target the upper body, to balance it with the lower body. Adding more shape and tone in the upper body will create the illusion of slimmer hips and thighs. You also need to do long-duration cardio work to shift that stubborn fat. The interval training programme suggested in the weekly exercise plan on page 137 will enable you to keep going for longer to achieve maximum results.

Recommended Rosemary Conley DVD:

Gi Jeans Weight-Loss Workout

Not only does this fitness DVD contain a long-duration aerobic workout and a salsa routine for optimum fat-burning, there's also plenty of toning work. Pick out the hip and thigh toning section so you can focus on your main problem area but don't forget also to do the upper body work from the Pear Shape Body Workout on the following pages to balance your whole body shape.

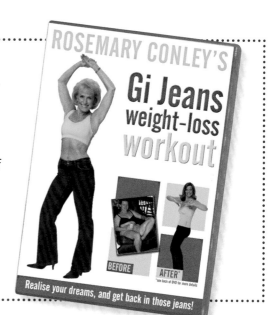

The Pear Shape Toning Workout with weights

For your weights use ½ litre bottles of water or ½–1kg handweights.

Warm-up

Warm up before you begin. Go for a 5-minute walk or march on the spot for 3 minutes, rotating your shoulders 10 times as you go Ⓐ. Lift your knees a little higher after 20 steps Ⓑ. Next, take 2 steps sideways Ⓒ to the left and then to the right. Repeat 4 times and then finish with a few gentle squats Ⓓ.

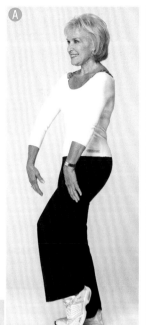

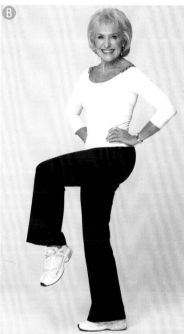

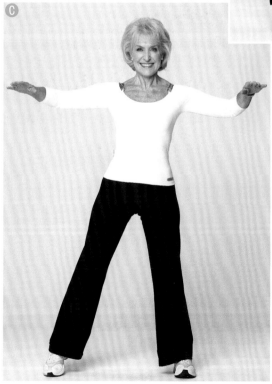

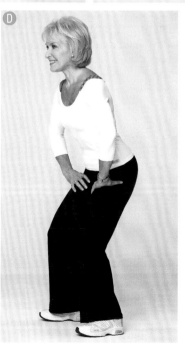

Toning programme

1 Hip and thigh toner with chest shaper

Take your legs out wide with your feet turned out slightly. Holding a handweight in each hand and your elbows out at shoulder height, lift the weights Ⓐ. Bend your knees, keeping your body upright, and bring your forearms together in front Ⓑ, then come up and open your arms out again.

Beginners: Do 1 to 2 sets of 8 reps
Intermediate: Do 3 to 4 sets of 10 reps

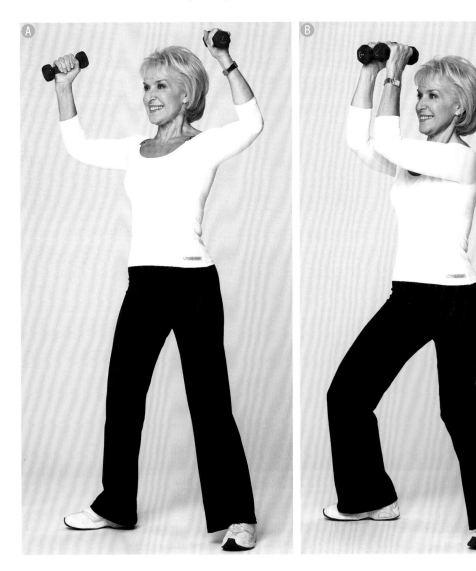

2 Bottom lifter with front of shoulder shaper

Stand with feet parallel and hip-width apart, a weight in each hand and your hands resting on your thighs Ⓐ. Pull your tummy in tight and lean forwards, lifting one leg behind, with toes forwards, and simultaneously bring your arms up to shoulder height, keeping your arms almost straight Ⓑ. Breathe out as you lift and in as you lower. Repeat, lifting the other leg, and keep repeating with alternate legs.

Beginners: Do 1 to 2 sets of 8 reps
Intermediate: Do 3 to 4 sets of 10 reps

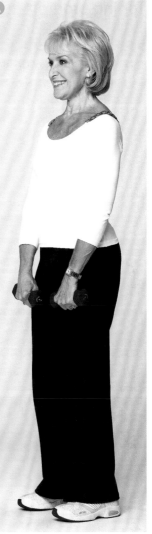

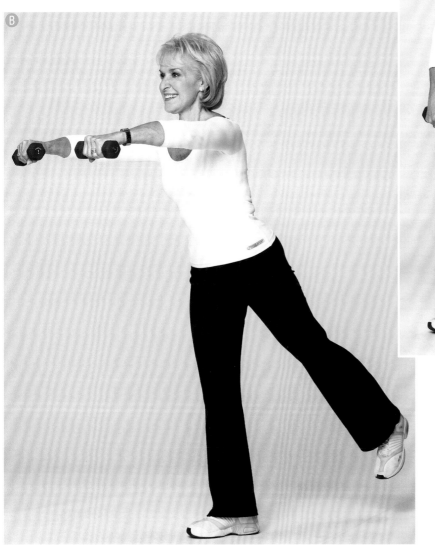

3 Outer thigh and top of shoulder shaper

Stand with feet hip-width apart and a weight in each hand Ⓐ. Lift both arms out to shoulder height and, as you do so, lift one leg out to the side, with toes forwards Ⓑ. Hold your tummy in to help you balance. Lower your arms and leg and repeat, lifting the other leg. Keep repeating with alternate legs, making sure your body stays upright and your knees and elbows slightly bent at all times.

Beginners: Do 1 to 2 sets of 8 reps
Intermediate: Do 3 to 4 sets of 10 reps

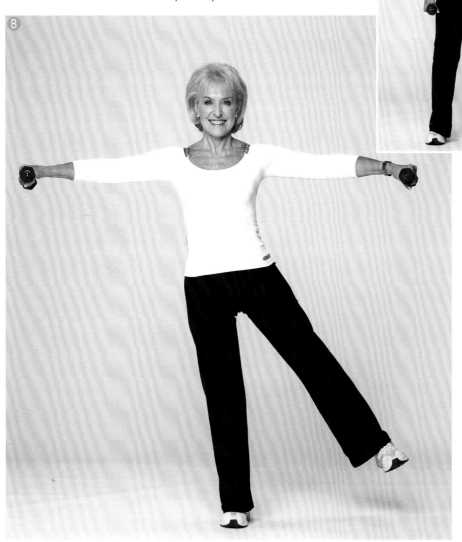

4 Thigh toner with bicep curl

Start with one foot a large step ahead of the other and stay on the ball of the back foot. Hold a weight in each hand Ⓐ. Keep your weight centred between both legs and hold your tummy in tight. Now bend both knees and, at the same time, bring your hands up to meet your shoulders Ⓑ. Come up again, straightening your legs and arms, then change legs and repeat. Keep repeating with alternate legs.

Beginners: Do 1 to 2 sets of 8 reps
Intermediate: Do 3 to 4 sets of 10 reps

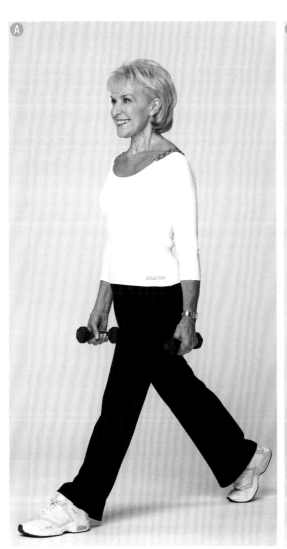

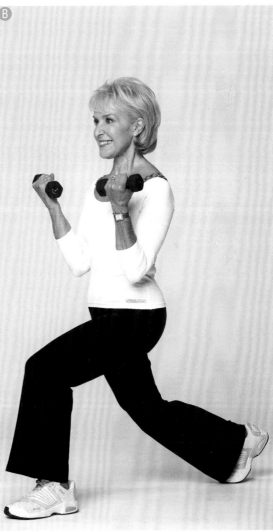

5 Tummy flattener with inner thigh toner

Lie on your back with knees bent and place a cushion between your knees Ⓐ. With hands behind your head, pull your tummy in tight and lift your head and shoulders off the floor, keeping your chin off your chest, and at the same time squeeze the cushion to work the inner thighs and the tummy Ⓑ. Breathe out as you lift and squeeze, and breathe in as you release and lower.

Beginners: Do 1 to 2 sets of 8 reps
Intermediate: Do 3 to 4 sets of 10 reps

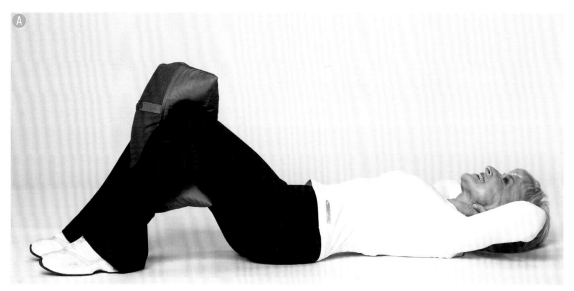

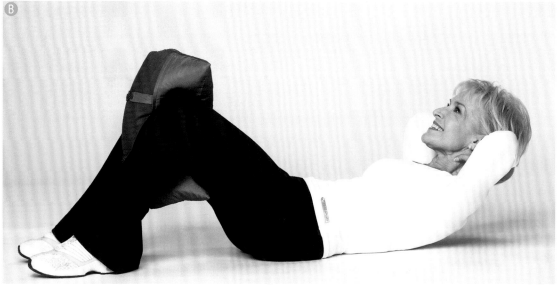

6 Chest and underarm toner

Come up onto your hands and knees, with knees directly under your hips (or slightly further back, which makes it harder) and wrists in line with your shoulders Ⓐ. Lower your upper body towards the floor, bending both elbows and taking your forehead in front of your fingers Ⓑ. Push up to straighten your elbows again, but without locking them out fully. Breathe in as you lower and breathe out as you lift.

Beginners: Do 1 to 2 sets of 8 reps
Intermediate: Do 3 to 4 sets of 10 reps

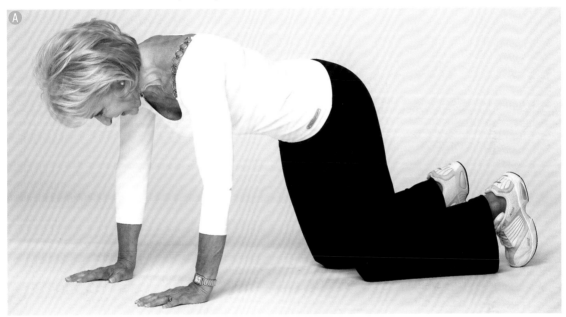

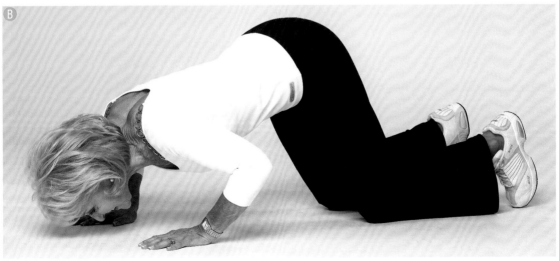

7 Tummy flattener with thigh toner

Lie on your back with knees bent, feet and knees together and hands behind your head Ⓐ. Lift your head and shoulders off the floor, keeping your chin off your chest and your tummy held in tight, and, at the same time, extend one leg straight, keeping your knees together Ⓑ. Lower again under control and repeat, lifting the other leg. Keep alternating legs.

Beginners: Do 1 to 2 sets of 8 reps
Intermediate: Do 3 to 4 sets of 10 reps

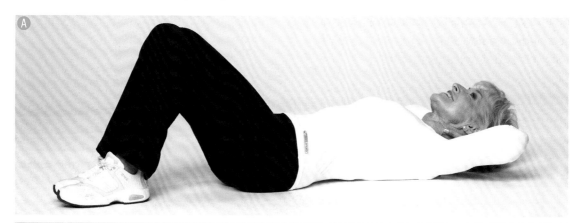

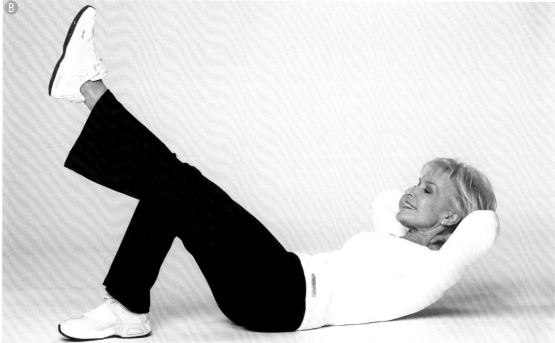

Now turn to page 134 to do your post-workout stretches.

The Pear Shape Toning Workout with resistance band

Warm-up

Warm up for 5 minutes by walking or marching, rolling your shoulders 10 times as you go Ⓐ. Lift your knees higher after 20 steps Ⓑ. Then do 8 sets of double side-steps Ⓒ followed by 8 simple squats Ⓓ.

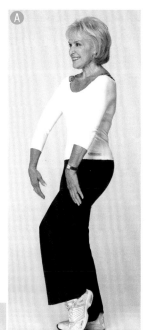

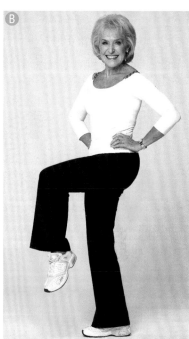

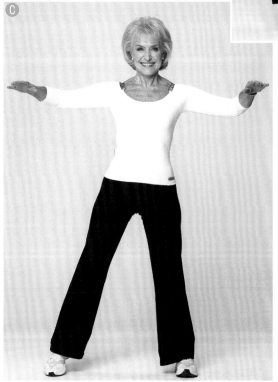

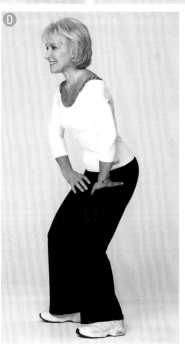

Toning programme

1 Hip and thigh toner with shoulder shaper
Stand with feet wider than your hips and turned out slightly. Place the band around your upper back and hold it at shoulder level Ⓐ. Squat down and as you bend your knees in line with your feet, push your arms overhead and slightly in front of you Ⓑ. Straighten your legs and bend your elbows to return to the start position. Keep your tummy in and stay upright without leaning forwards or back.
Beginners: Do 1 to 2 sets of 12 reps
Intermediate: Do 3 to 4 sets of 12 reps

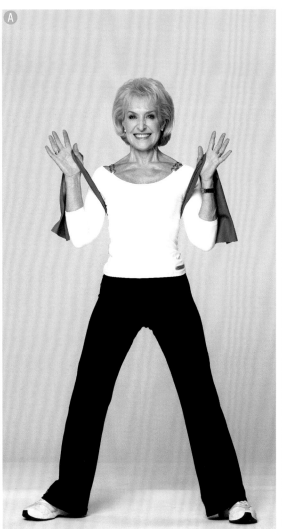

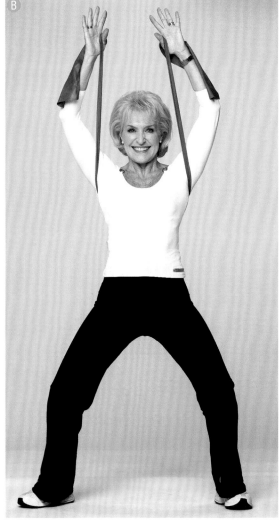

2 Hip and thigh toner with underarm firmer

Stand with feet parallel and slightly wider than your hips. Position the band across your hips, with hands on your hips and elbows pointing back. Pull your tummy in and lean forwards Ⓐ. Bend your knees in line with your feet and, at the same time, push your hips back and almost straighten your elbows behind you Ⓑ. Bend your elbows again and straighten your legs to return to the start position.

Beginners: Do 1 to 2 sets of 8 reps
Intermediate: Do 3 to 4 sets of 10 reps

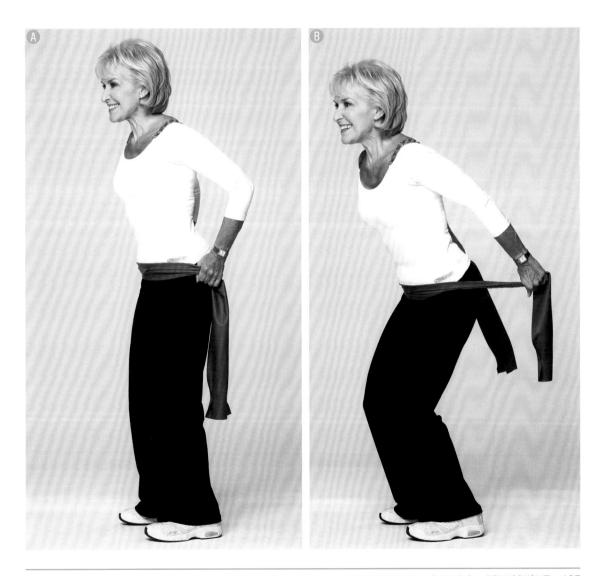

3 Tummy toner with chest shaper

Lie on your back with knees bent and the band placed under your shoulder blades and armpits. Grip the band between your thumb and forefinger (A). Pull your tummy in tight and, as you curl your upper body off the floor, keeping your chin off your chest, extend your arms towards your knees (B), then lower again. Breathe out as you lift and breathe in as you lower.

Beginners: Do 1 to 2 sets of 8 reps
Intermediate: Do 3 to 4 sets of 10 reps

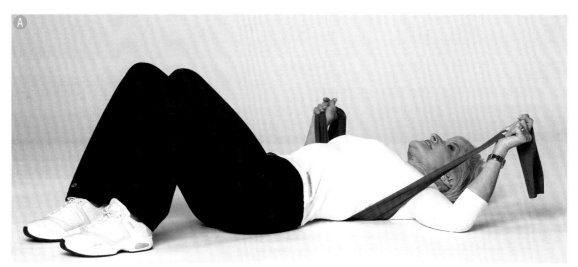

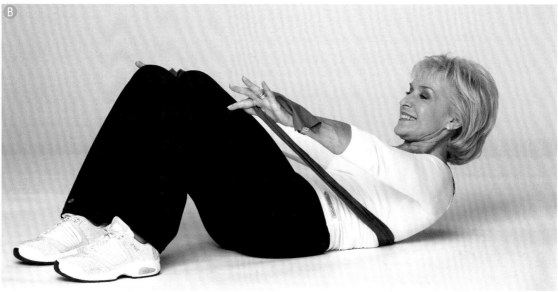

4 Bottom shaper

Lie on your back with knees bent and the band placed across your hips. Secure the band on the floor with your hands. Bring your left ankle on top of your right knee Ⓐ. (You can keep your feet on the floor if you find this uncomfortable.) Now, keeping your tummy pulled in tight, lift your hips off the floor, without arching your back, and squeeze your buttocks together while keeping the band firmly on the floor Ⓑ. Lower again, then lift and lower for a full set of reps before changing legs and repeating.

Beginners: Do 1 to 2 sets of 12 reps on each side
Intermediate: Do 3 to 4 sets of 12 reps on each side

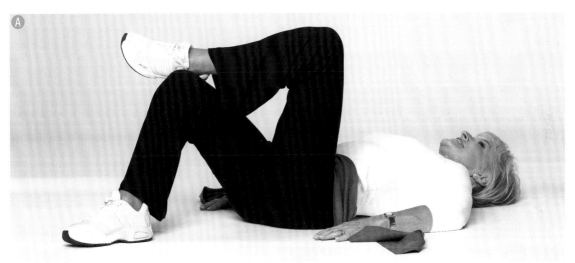

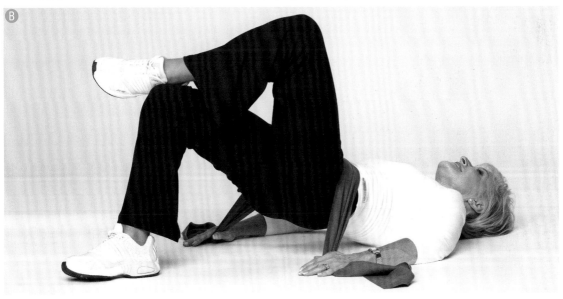

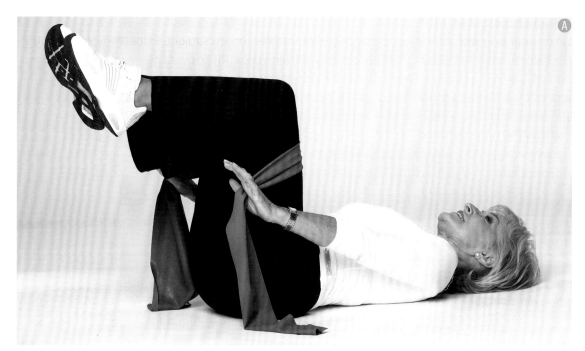

5 Tummy flattener

Lie on your back with your legs up at a 90-degree angle, legs together, and place the band across your thighs Ⓐ. Lift your head and shoulders off the floor, keeping a gap between your chin and chest, and push the band away from you Ⓑ. Breathe out as you lift and in as you lower.

Beginners: Do 1 to 2 sets of 8 reps

Intermediate: Do 3 to 4 sets of 10 reps

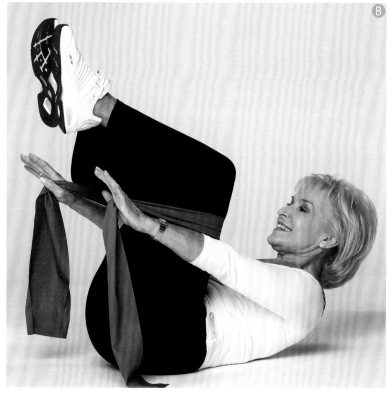

6 Two-stage outer thigh shaper

Lie on your side with your lower leg slightly bent and the top leg straight. Place the band over your thighs then wrap it around to the front again, allowing the ends to overlap. Hold the ends of the band in one hand and rest your head on the other hand Ⓐ. Keeping the foot of the straight leg facing forwards, not up, lift the leg and stop halfway Ⓑ and then lift further, keeping the leg straight and without dropping your hips forwards or back Ⓒ. Lower under control, again stopping halfway through the range. Do a full set of reps on one side, then repeat on the other side.

Beginners: Do 1 to 2 sets of 8 reps on each side
Intermediate: Do 3 to 4 sets of 10 reps on each side

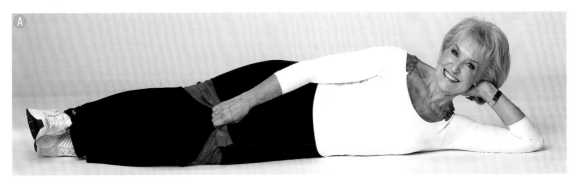

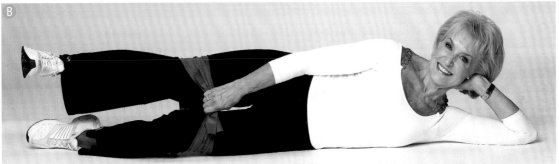

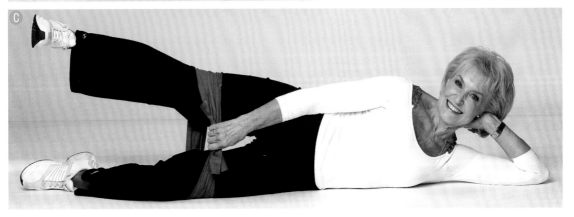

7 Inner thigh toner

Lie on your side with your top knee bent and resting on a rolled-up towel, with the underneath leg extended and straight Ⓐ. Lift the underneath leg, keeping it straight Ⓑ, and as you lower it try not to touch the floor. Do a full set of reps with one leg, then turn over and repeat with the other leg.

Beginners: Do 1 to 2 sets of 8 reps on each leg
Intermediate: Do 3 to 4 sets of 10 reps on each leg

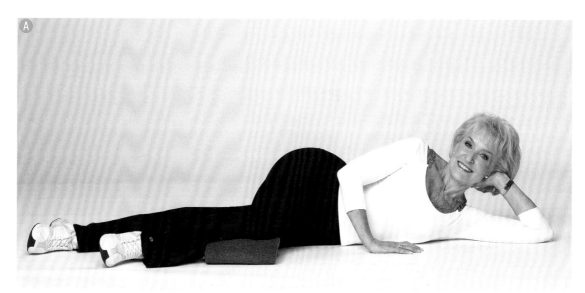

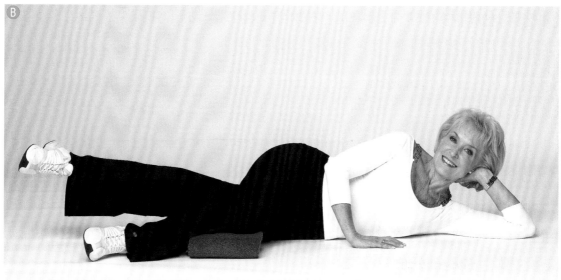

8 Chest and underarm shaper

Come up onto your hands and knees, with knees directly under your hips (or slightly further back, which makes it harder) and wrists in line with your shoulders. Place the band over your shoulder blades and secure it on the floor with your hands Ⓐ. With fingers facing forwards, bend both elbows and take your forehead in front of your fingers Ⓑ. Now push up to almost straighten the elbows again, but without locking them out fully. Breathe in as you lower and breathe out as you lift.

Beginners: Do 1 to 2 sets of 8 reps
Intermediate: Do 3 to 4 sets of 10 reps

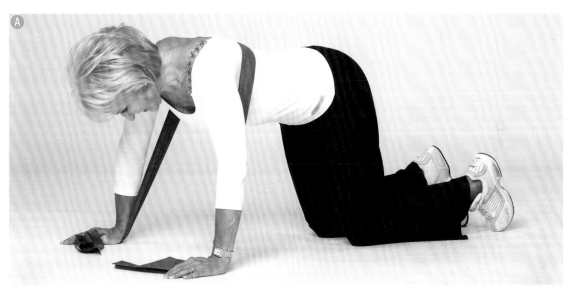

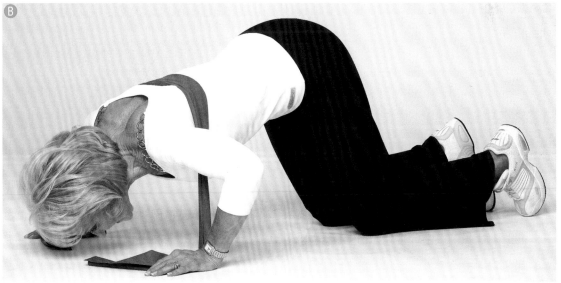

Now finish your workout with the stretches below.

Post-Workout Stretches

1 Front of thigh stretch

Lie on your front, bend one knee and hold it with the same-side hand. Rest your head on the other hand, relax your upper body and bring your knees together, pressing the hips into the floor. Hold for 10 seconds, then change legs and repeat.

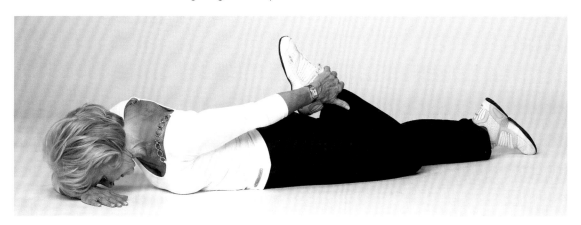

2 Tummy stretch

Still lying on your front, place your bent forearms out to the sides, with your elbows in line with your shoulders. Now lift your head and shoulders off the floor to prop yourself up on your elbows and lift your chin slightly to feel a stretch down the abdominal area. Hold for 10 seconds, then release.

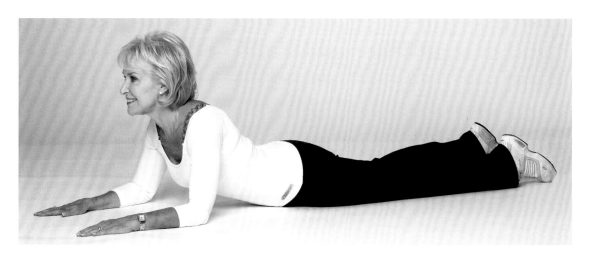

3 Chest stretch

Sit upright and bring both arms behind you on the floor. Bring your shoulder blades together behind your back to feel a stretch in the chest muscles. Hold for 10 seconds, then release.

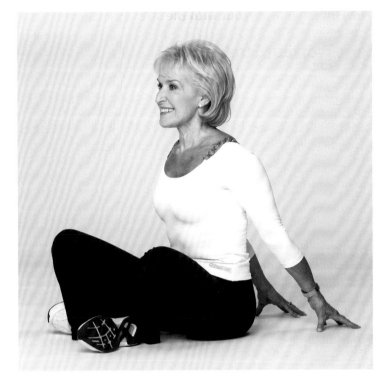

4 Inner thigh stretch

Sit with the soles of your feet together, hands around your ankles and elbows resting inside your knees. Sit up straight and then lean forwards slightly. Keeping your back straight, gently press your knees further apart with your elbows to stretch your inner thighs. Hold for 10 seconds, then breathe in and, as you breathe out, press your knees down further to slightly increase the stretch for another 10 seconds.

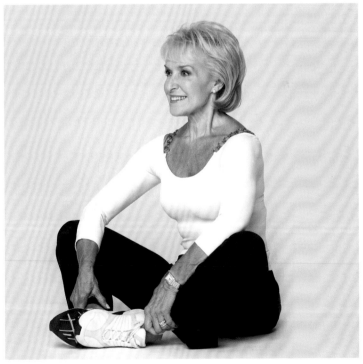

5 Outer thigh and hip stretch

Extend both legs out in front, then bring your left foot across the right knee. Place your right hand on your left knee. Now lift your body upright and ease the left knee across your body to feel a stretch in the left outer thigh and hip. Hold for 10 seconds, then change legs and repeat.

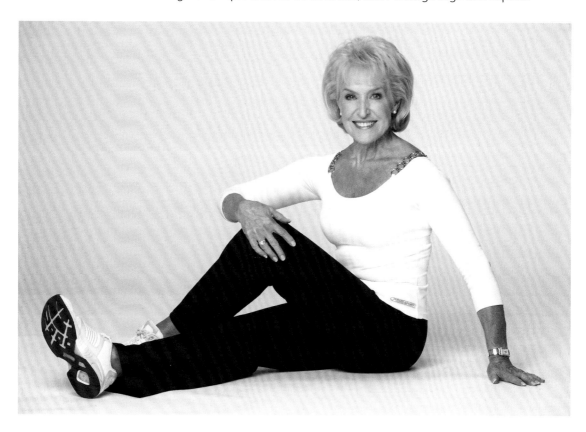

Pear Shape Weekly Exercise Plan

Day	Type	Beginners	Intermediate
1	Cardio interval training	Gentle walk 3 mins Power walk 4 mins Repeat twice	Power walk 5 mins Gentle jog 5 mins Repeat 3 times for a 30-minute workout
2	Pear Shape Toning Workout		Pear Shape Toning Workout
3	Cardio interval training	Swim, cycle or cross-trainer 20 mins *OR* Do DVD whole programme	Swim breaststroke 5 mins Fast front crawl 5 mins Repeat 3 times for a 30-minute workout
4	Cardio interval training	Gentle walk 2 mins Power walk 5 mins Repeat 3 times	Power walk 5 mins Gentle jog 5 mins Repeat 3 times for a 30-minute workout
5	Pear Shape Toning Workout		Pear Shape Toning Workout
6	Cardio/tone	Swim, cycle or cross-trainer 20 mins *OR* Do DVD whole programme	Do DVD at intermediate or high level *OR* Swim or walk/jog 40 mins + Pear Shape Toning Workout
7	Cardio/tone	Walk, swim or cycle 30 mins + Pear Shape Toning Workout	Swim breaststroke 5 mins Fast front crawl 5 mins Repeat 3 times for a 30-minute workout *OR* Cycle, jog or cross-trainer 30 mins + Pear Shape Toning Workout

MONITOR YOUR PROGRESS

	Weight	BMI	Waist-to-hip ratio
Start			
End month 1			
End month 2			
End month 3			
End month 4			

Post-Cardio Stretches

Learn the following stretches so that you can do them after every walk or cardio workout. They will stretch out the leg muscles that you've worked hard and prevent you from aching later.

1 Calf stretch

Stand with one foot in front of the other, with both feet pointing forwards. Bend the front knee in line with the ankle and have the back foot as far back as possible to feel a strong stretch in the calf. Hold for 10 seconds, then release. Change legs and repeat.

2 Lower calf and chest stretch

Stand upright with one foot slightly ahead of the other, feet hip-width apart and both knees bent, to feel a stretch in the lower calf. At the same time, take both hands behind you and open your shoulders to feel a stretch across the chest. Hold for 10 seconds, then release. Change legs and repeat.

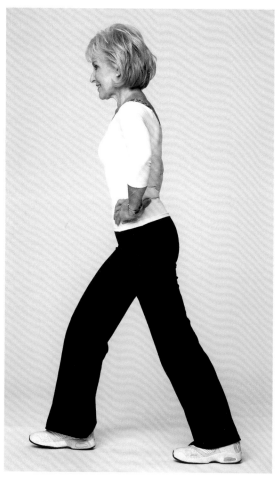 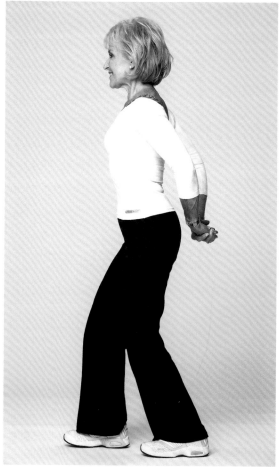

3 Front of hip stretch

Take your right leg behind you and stay on the ball of the foot. Now bend both knees and push your right hip further forwards to feel a stretch at the front of that hip. Keep your body straight and directly above your hips. Hold for 10 seconds, then release. Change legs and repeat.

4 Front of thigh stretch

Stand tall and take hold of one ankle, using a chair or wall for support if necessary. Make sure your knees are in line with each other and the standing leg is slightly bent. Hold for 10 seconds, then release. Change legs and repeat.

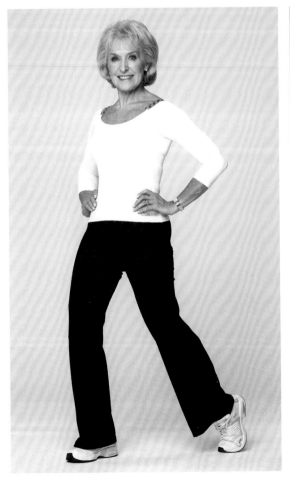

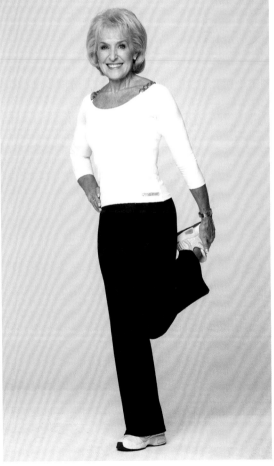

5 Inner thigh stretch

Stand with your legs wide and your feet turned out slightly. Now bend your left leg, keeping the knee in line with the ankle, and turn your right foot to point forwards with your right leg straight, taking it far enough away from your left leg to feel a stretch in the inner thigh of the right leg. Hold for 10 seconds, then release. Change legs and repeat.

6 Back of thigh and hip stretch

Stand with one leg in front of the other, feet hip-width apart, with the front leg straight and the back leg bent. Lean forwards slightly, keeping your back straight and your head in line with your spine. Lift your hips up to feel a stretch in the back of the thigh and the hip of the front leg. Hold for 10 seconds, then release. Change legs and repeat.

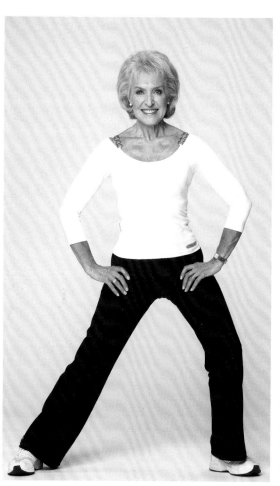

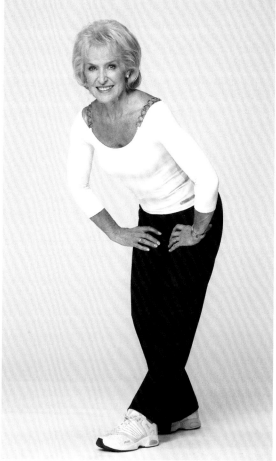

18
The Stay Young Apple Shape Workout

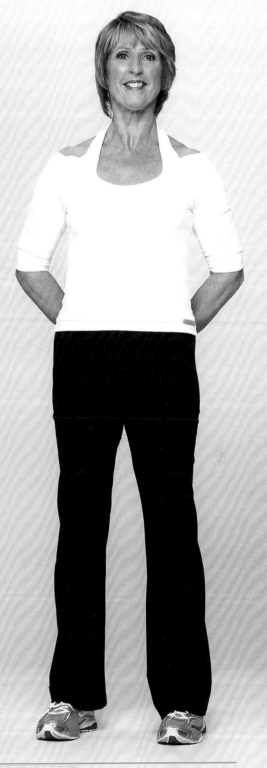

If you are apple-shaped, your top half will be bigger than your more slender lower half. You will probably have enviably slim legs and arms, which will stay looking slim for ever and you're unlikely to ever suffer from batwings. Lucky you! While you may envy a pear shape's slim waist, they would swap it for your arms and legs any day!

As an apple shape, you will tend to gather your fat around your middle, particularly on your tummy and, if you gain weight, it will go straight there! You'll also find you have a flattish bottom, which may become flatter as you get older unless you work at keeping it in shape. Also, your legs may become too thin, compared to your trunk, so you need to strengthen your legs by doing some good muscle-toning and strength exercises to maintain their lovely shape. And you can tone that tummy and achieve a flat one if you're prepared to work at it. It's all very 'do-able' but, if you are to transform your shape, you have to *want* to do it.

My apple-shaped model is Mary Morris MSc, my fitness consultant who has worked alongside me for the last 16 years. Not only does Mary have an enviable body, she has also had three children, two of which were twins who weighed in at 7lb 1oz and 8lb at birth! So if Mary can have a flat stomach, anyone can.

Mary was one of the original team who created the Exercise to Music qualification in 1986, which has transformed the fitness industry. For 30 years Mary ran her own health and fitness club in Lichfield, Staffs, and she has spent her life helping others to become fitter through safe and effective exercise and activity. As a mature student, Mary graduated with a Masters degree in Exercise and Nutrition Science when she was 50. Mary is now in her early 60s.

The best exercise for your shape

Your weekly workout programme includes plenty of aerobic activity to help burn fat from all over your body but particularly your abdomen. The stronger your abs the better, as stronger muscles burn more fat, added to which you'll be able to hold your tummy in much more easily and effectively.

Walking, aerobics, running, swimming, using a stepper and working out on the cross-trainer will all make you fitter, but the bonus is that they will all work your bottom as well as your legs to keep you in great shape for ever.

This toning workout focuses on tummy flattening, waist shrinking and bottom building as well as keeping your legs in good shape so that they don't become too thin as you get older. You need to do this workout at least three times a week for great results.

Recommended Rosemary Conley DVD:

Real Results Workout

Not only is there a bonus aerobic fat-burning session and plenty of toning work in this fitness DVD, but there's also a four-minute express abs workout, which is so quick and easy to do after your fat-burning sessions.

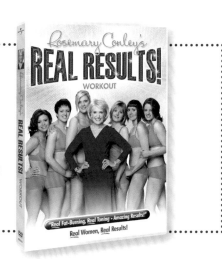

The Apple Shape Toning Workout with weights

For your weights use ½ litre bottles of water or ½–1kg handweights.

Warm-up

Warm up for 5 minutes before you begin. March on the spot, rolling your shoulders 10 times as you march for 2 minutes Ⓐ. Then, with feet hip-width apart and arms above your head Ⓑ, 'ski down' 8 times, bending your knees and swinging your arms down Ⓒ and then up again. Now do a twisted ski 8 times, bringing both arms down to alternate sides and up again as you bend your knees Ⓓ, keeping your tummy in tight to support your back.

continued…

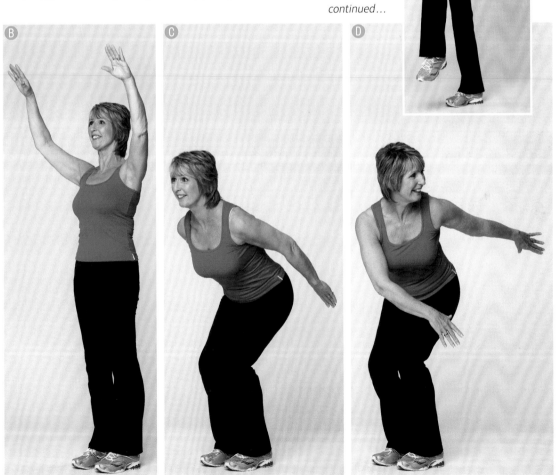

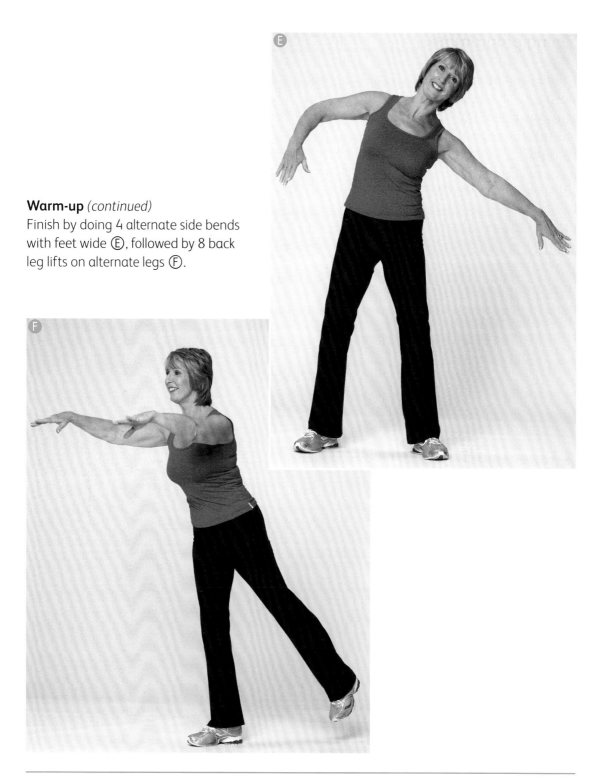

Warm-up *(continued)*
Finish by doing 4 alternate side bends with feet wide Ⓔ, followed by 8 back leg lifts on alternate legs Ⓕ.

Toning programme

1 Waist-toning side bend

Stand tall with feet just wider than your shoulders, a handweight in one hand and the other hand behind your head Ⓐ. Pull your tummy in tight and bend your trunk towards the weight, keeping your hips still and without leaning forwards or back Ⓑ. Return to the centre and repeat to the same side for a full set of reps, then change sides and repeat.

Beginners: Do 1 to 2 sets of 8 reps to each side
Intermediate: Do 3 to 4 sets of 10 reps to each side

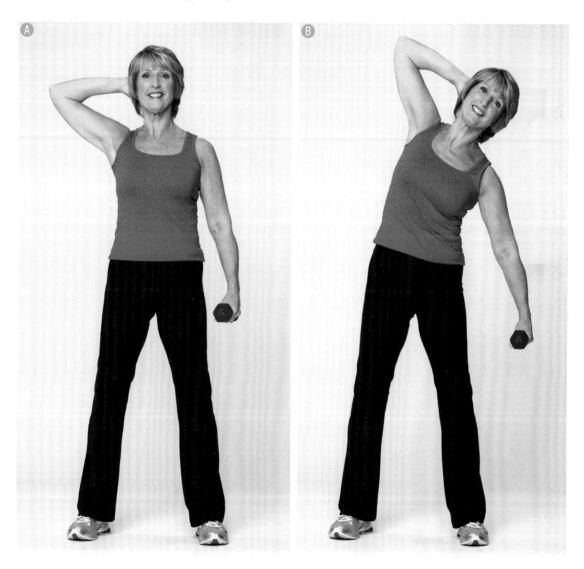

2 Twisted ski waist trimmer

Stand tall with feet hip-width apart, holding one weight in both hands and hands resting on your thighs. Lift the weight above your head, holding your tummy in, then without leaning back Ⓐ, twist your trunk and take the weight down to one side, bending your knees Ⓑ. Lift it above your head again and twist down to the other side. Keep repeating to alternate sides.

Beginners: Do 1 to 2 sets of 8 reps
Intermediate: Do 3 to 4 sets of 10 reps

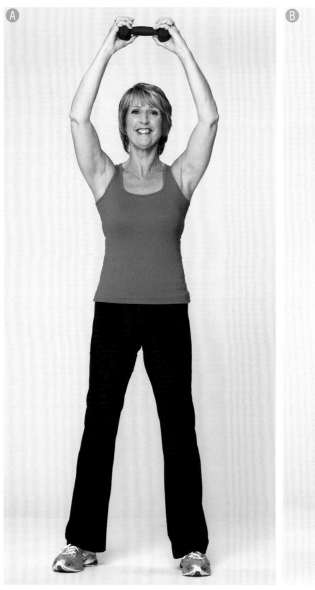

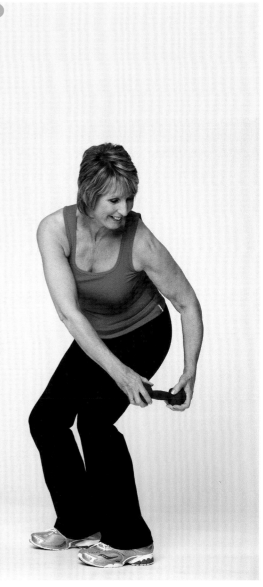

3 Bottom toner with shoulder shaper

Stand with feet parallel and hip-width apart, holding a weight in each hand and hands resting on your thighs Ⓐ. Pull your tummy in tight and lean forwards as you lift one leg behind and bring your straight arms up to chest height Ⓑ. Lower again and repeat on the other leg. Keep repeating on alternate legs. Breathe out as you lift and in as you lower.

Beginners: Do 1 to 2 sets of 8 reps
Intermediate: Do 3 to 4 sets of 10 reps

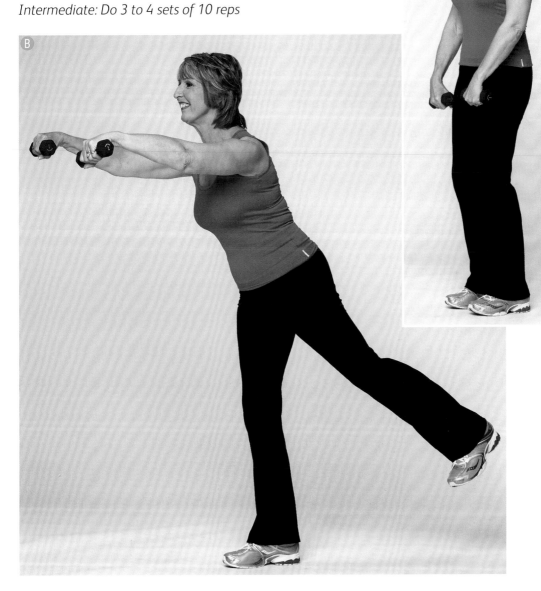

4 Tummy flattener

Lie on your back with knees bent, feet flat on the floor and hip-width apart. Place one hand behind your head and have the other hand reaching towards the same-side leg Ⓐ. Breathe in and, as you breathe out, pull your tummy in tight and lift your head and shoulders off the floor, keeping your chin off your chest Ⓑ, then lower. Do a full set of reps on one side and then change sides and repeat.

Beginners: Do 1 to 2 sets of 8 reps on each side
Intermediate: Do 3 to 4 sets of 10 reps on each side

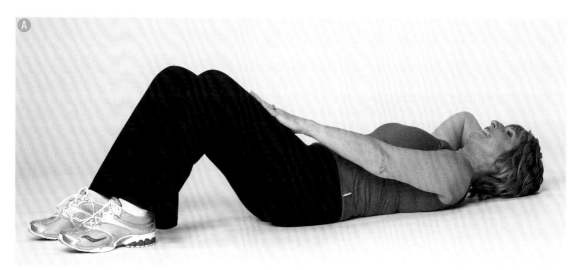

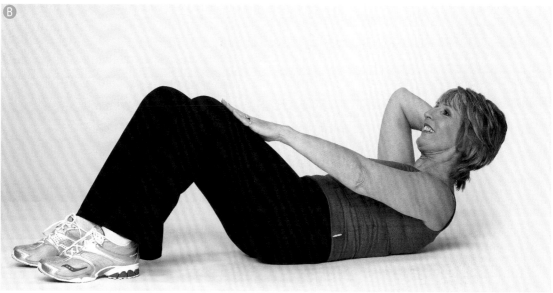

5 Waist-trimming twist with leg extension

Lie on your back with both knees bent, feet hip-width apart and both hands behind your head
Ⓐ. Lift your head and shoulders off the floor and twist your waist towards your left leg as you
slide the leg along the floor to extend fully Ⓑ. Lower again, sliding the leg back to the bent start
position. Repeat, twisting your waist to your right leg as you slide the right leg along the floor
and keep repeating to alternate sides. Breathe out as you lift and in as you lower.

Beginners: Do 1 to 2 sets of 8 reps to each side
Intermediate: Do 3 to 4 sets of 10 reps to each side

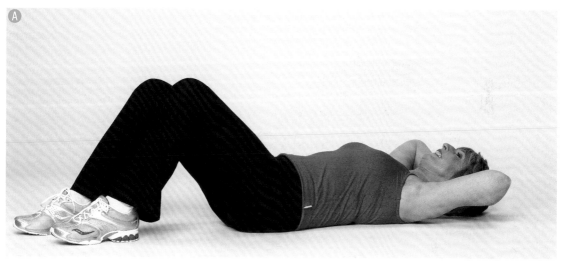

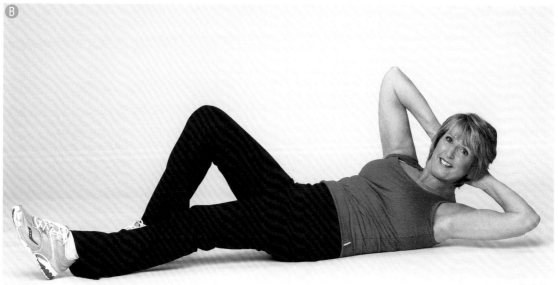

6 Tummy-flattening 'half' or 'full' plank

Come up onto your elbows and knees, with your head in line with your spine and your trunk flat Ⓐ. Alternatively, you can extend your legs and rest on your elbows and toes Ⓑ. Pull your tummy in very tight and hold for a maximum of 10 seconds. Breathe normally while holding your tummy in tight throughout. Release.

Beginners: Do a maximum of 4 times, holding for 10 seconds each time

Intermediate: Do 4 times but hold for 20 seconds each time

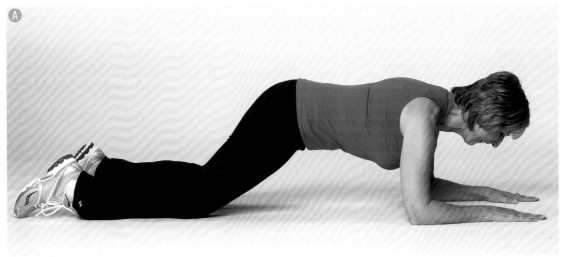

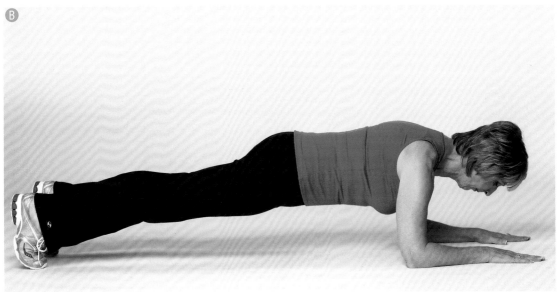

7 Tummy-tightening and back-strengthening table top

Come up onto your hands and knees, with hands directly under your shoulders and knees under your hips. Pull your tummy in to support your back and straighten your right leg out behind, keeping the foot in contact with the floor Ⓐ. Now lift your right foot off the floor and, at the same time, lift your left arm out in line with your ear Ⓑ. Hold for 2 seconds, find your balance and then slowly lower. Change sides and repeat.

Beginners: Do 1 to 2 sets of 8 reps (4 to each side)
Intermediate: Do 3 to 4 sets of 10 reps (5 to each side)

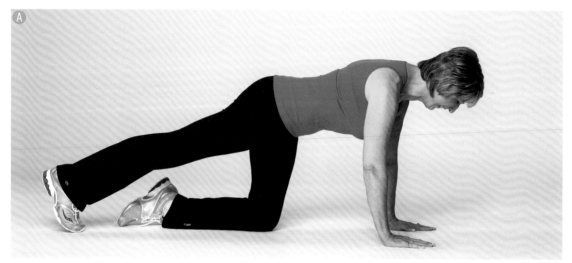

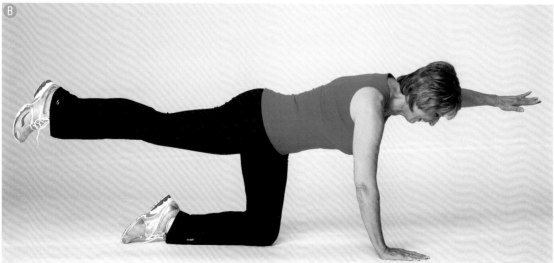

Now turn to page 161 to do your post-workout stretches.

The Apple Shape Toning Workout with resistance band

Warm-up

Warm up for 5 minutes by marching on the spot for 2 minutes, rotating your shoulders 10 times as you march Ⓐ. Then take your feet wide and bend to alternate sides 8 times Ⓑ. Now stand tall and ski down 8 times Ⓒ, bending your knees and swinging your arms down and then up again Ⓓ.

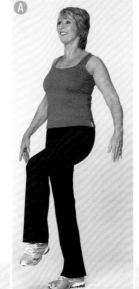

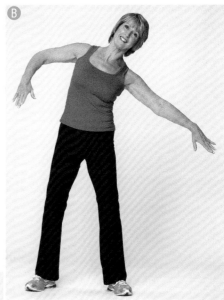

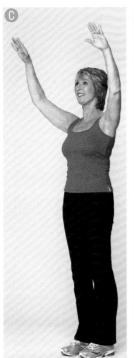

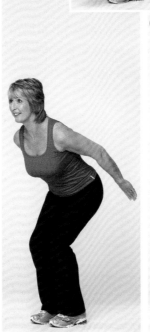

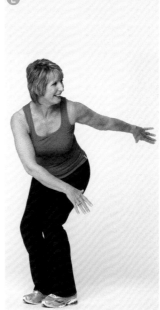

Finish with 8 twisted skis, bringing both arms down to alternate sides and then up again as you bend your knees Ⓔ.

Toning programme

1 Thigh-toning squat

Stand in the middle of the band, with your feet hip-width apart and the band pulled up to hip height Ⓐ. Bend your knees in line with your feet, pushing your hips back and keeping your spine in a straight line with your head Ⓑ. Your weight should be more in the heels. As you lift up again try not to lock out the knees.

Beginners: Do 1 to 2 sets of 8 reps
Intermediate: Do 3 to 4 sets of 10 reps

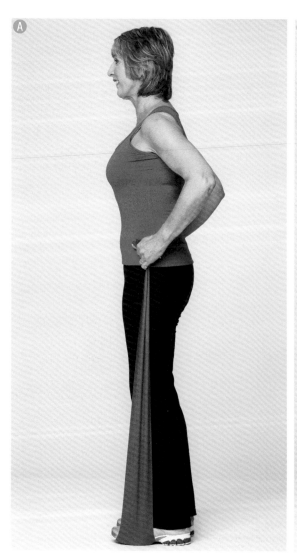

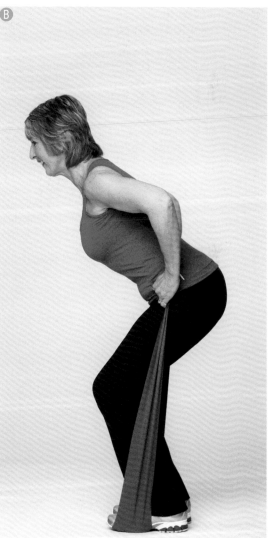

2 Tummy-flattening curl-ups

Lie on your back with knees bent and the band wrapped around your thighs, just above your knees. Hold both ends in one hand and place your other hand behind your head Ⓐ. Now pull your tummy in tight and lift your head and shoulders off the floor, keeping your chin off your chest and pulling on the band for a greater lift Ⓑ. Lower again and repeat, breathing out as you lift and in as you lower.

Beginners: Do 2 sets of 8 reps
Intermediate: See advanced exercise opposite

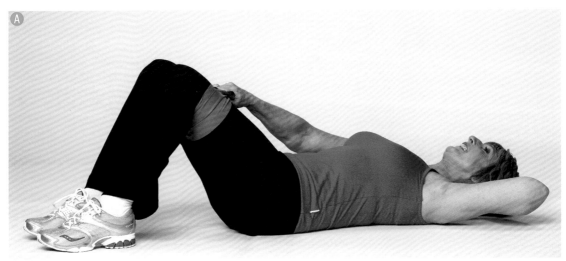

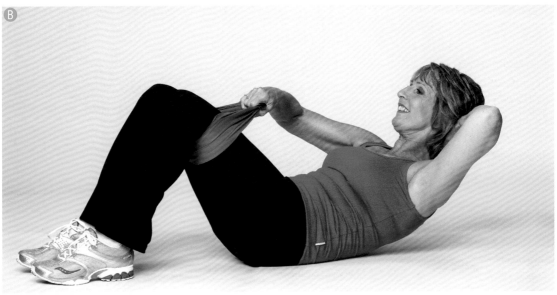

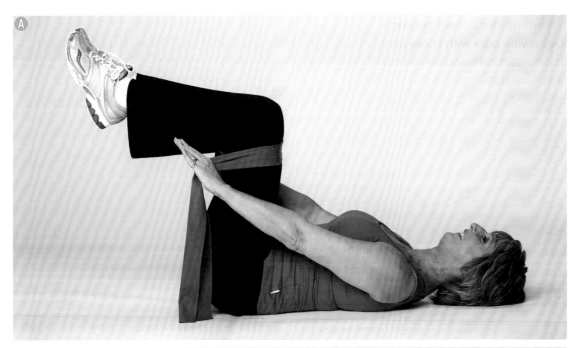

3 Super-flattening advanced abdominal crunch

Lie on your back with your legs up at a 90-degree angle, legs together, and the band placed flat across your lower thighs Ⓐ. Lift your head and shoulders off the floor and, at the same time, push the band away, keeping a gap between your chin and chest, and lift your hips just off the floor Ⓑ. Breathe out as you lift and in as you lower.

Intermediate only:
Do 2 to 3 sets of 8 reps

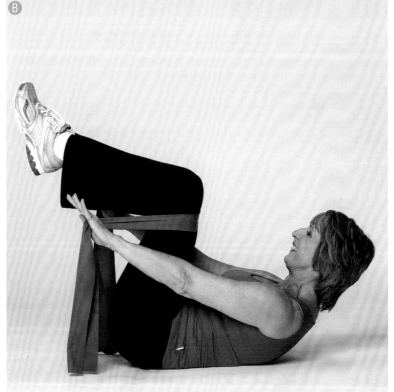

4 Waist-shrinking twist

Lie on your back with the band under your shoulder blades and armpits and your left hand behind your head Ⓐ. Now pull your tummy in tight as you lift your head and shoulders off the floor, and reach your right hand across to the left knee Ⓑ. Breathe in before you lift and then breathe out as you lift up and across. Keep repeating on the same side for a full set of reps and then change sides and repeat.

Beginners: Do 2 sets of 8 reps to each side
Intermediate: see advanced exercise opposite

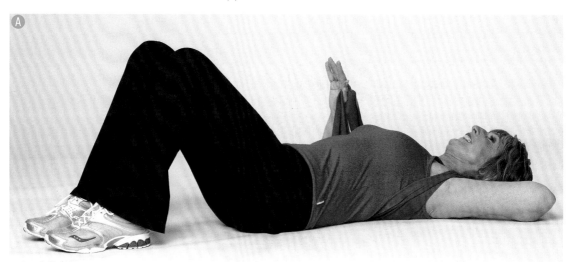

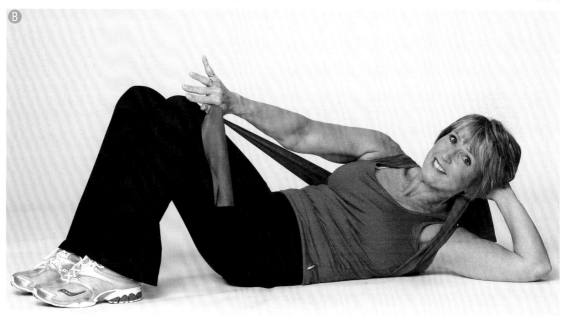

5 Advanced waist-shrinking twist

Lie on your back with your hands behind your head and both knees bent and off the floor Ⓐ. Pull your tummy in tight and lift your head and shoulders off the floor, twisting your right shoulder to your bent left leg as you extend your left leg out to 45 degrees Ⓑ. Keeping your head and shoulders off the floor, change from side to side for a full set of reps, then rest before repeating further sets.

Intermediate only: Do 2 to 3 sets of 8 reps

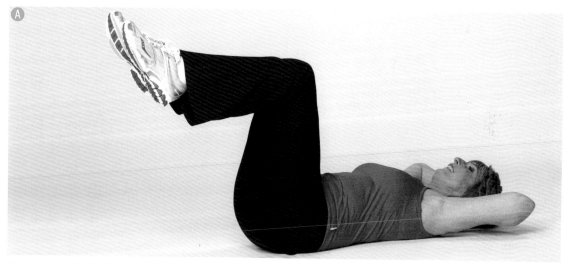

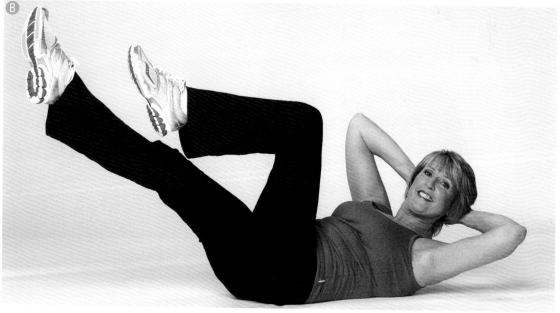

6 Bottom-shaper hip raise

Lie on your back with your legs bent. Place the band across your hips and secure it on the floor with your hands. Bring your left ankle on top of your right knee Ⓐ. (Alternatively, keep both feet on the floor.) Now lift your hips off the floor without arching your back but keep the band firmly on the floor Ⓑ. Lower again, then lift and lower for a full set of reps before changing legs.

Beginners: Do 1 set of 12 reps on each leg
Intermediate: Do 2 sets of 12 reps on each leg

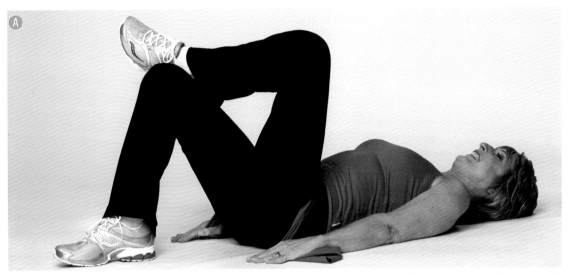

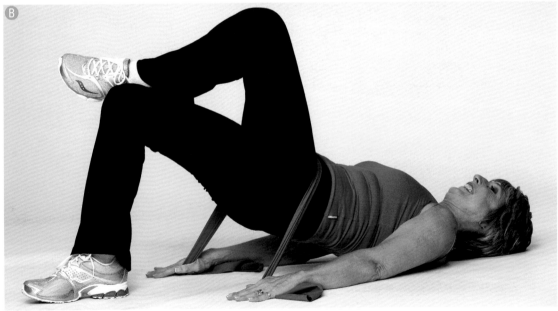

7 Oyster with leg raise waist toner

Lie on your side with your head resting on your hand, both knees bent to 45 degrees and the band wrapped around both legs, just above knees Ⓐ. Your feet should be in line with your hips and shoulders. Start by pulling your tummy in so that your waist lifts from the floor. Now lift the top knee to open your knees Ⓑ, then lift both feet off the floor, keeping your feet together, knees apart and without dropping your hips back Ⓒ. Lower again with control. Do a full set of reps on this side, then change sides and repeat.

Beginners: Do 1 to 2 sets of 8 reps on each side
Intermediate: Do 3 to 4 sets of 10 reps on each side

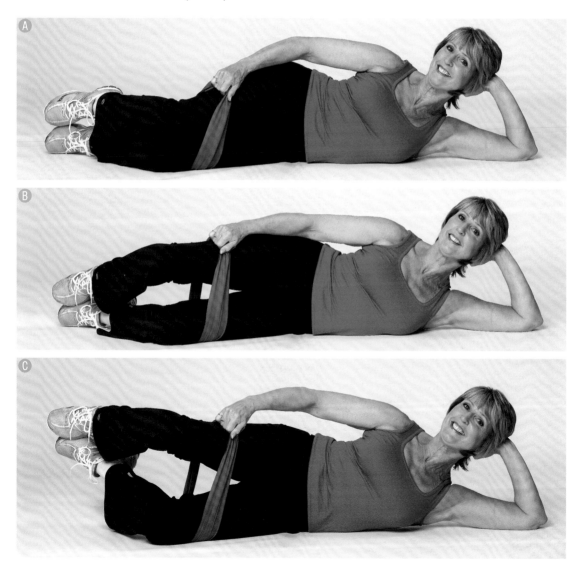

8 Spine strengthener and waist trimmer

Lie on your front with the band placed across your upper back and secured on the floor with both hands. Keep your legs together and rest your forehead on a folded towel Ⓐ. Pull your tummy in and lift your head off the towel while pushing your arms out to the sides in line with your shoulders Ⓑ. Bend your spine down the right side to work your waist Ⓒ. Keep facing the floor at all times. Come back to the centre and rest your forehead on the towel before repeating on the other side.

Beginners: Do 1 set of 6 reps to each side
Intermediate: Do 2 sets of 6 reps to each side

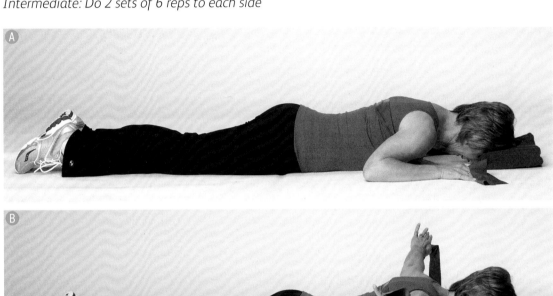

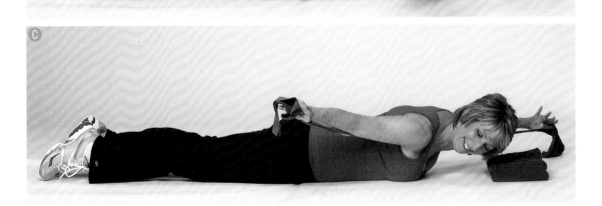

Finish with the stretches below.

Post-Workout Stretches

1 Abdominal stretch

Lie on your front and place your forearms out to the sides, with your elbows in line with your shoulders. Now lift your head and shoulders off the floor to prop yourself up on your elbows and lift your chin slightly to feel a stretch down your tummy. Hold for 10 seconds, then release.

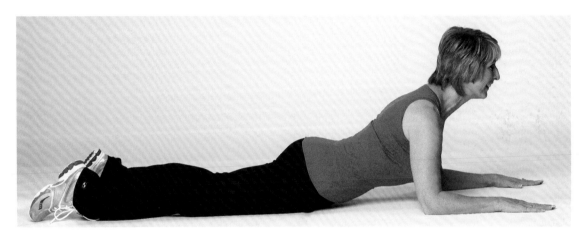

2 Spine stretch

Now come up onto your hands and knees and pull your tummy in as you arch your spine up towards the ceiling. Draw your head down to look at your tummy and keep your shoulders down, away from your ears, and your neck relaxed. Hold for 10 seconds, then release.

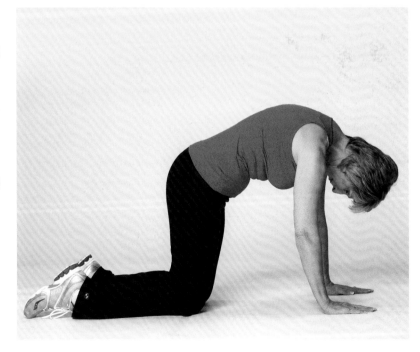

3 Waist stretch

Sit up with legs crossed and reach your right arm up overhead. Now, keeping both hips firmly on the floor, lean to the left to feel a stretch in the waist on your right side. Try not to lean forwards or back. Hold for 10 seconds, then release. Change sides and repeat.

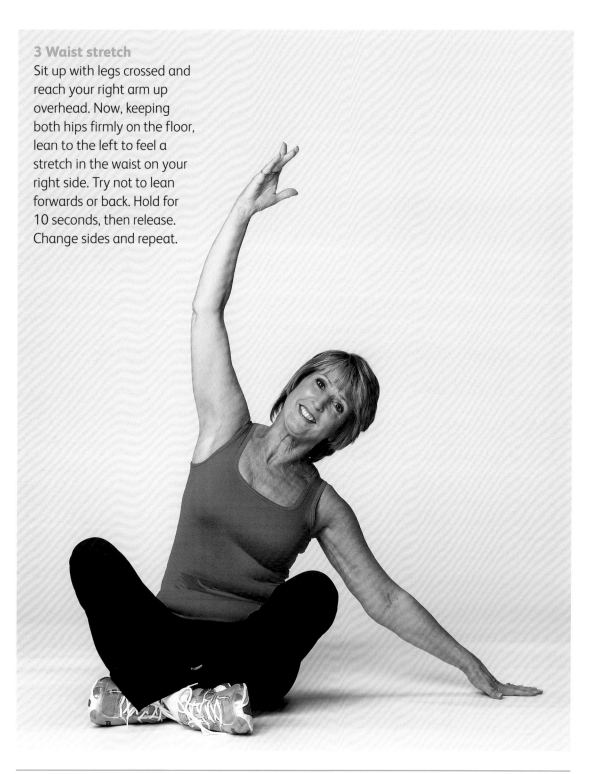

Apple Shape Weekly Exercise Plan

Day	Type	Beginners	Intermediate
1	Cardio/tone	Walk 15 mins at a moderate pace + 20 tummy curls	Power walk 5 mins Gentle jog 2 mins Repeat 3 times for a workout time of just over 20 mins + 2 sets × 15 tummy curls
2	Apple Shape Toning Workout		Apple Shape Toning Workout
3	Cardio/tone	Walk, swim or cycle 20 mins + Apple Shape Toning Workout	Power walk, cycle or cross-trainer 30 mins + Apple Shape Toning Workout
4	Cardio/tone	Walk 20 mins at a brisk pace + 20 tummy curls	Mix swim, cycle or cross-trainer 30 mins + 5 tummy curls and 15 waist twists
5	Apple Shape Toning Workout		Apple Shape Toning Workout
6	Cardio/tone	Do DVD whole programme at beginner level OR Power Walk 20 mins + Apple Shape Toning Workout	Do DVD whole programme at intermediate or high level OR Swim or power walk 40 mins + Apple Shape Toning Workout
7	Cardio/tone	Walk, swim or cycle 30 mins + 20 tummy curls	Power walk 5 mins Gentle jog 3 mins Do 3 times for a workout time of just under 25 mins + 2 sets × 15 tummy curls

MONITOR YOUR PROGRESS

	Weight	BMI	Waist-to-hip ratio
Start			
End month 1			
End month 2			
End month 3			
End month 4			

Post-Cardio Stretches

Learn these stretches so that they can be done after every aerobic activity. They will help to keep your muscles extended and prevent aching later.

1 Calf stretch
Stand with one foot in front of the other and both feet pointing forwards. Bend your front knee in line with the ankle, keeping your back foot as far back as possible to feel a strong stretch in the calf. Hold for 10 seconds, then release. Change legs and repeat.

2 Lower calf and chest stretch
Stand upright with one foot slightly ahead of the other and feet a hip-width apart. Bend both knees to feel a stretch in the lower calf of the back leg. At the same time, take both hands behind you and open your shoulders to feel a stretch across your chest. Hold for 10 seconds, then release. Change legs and repeat.

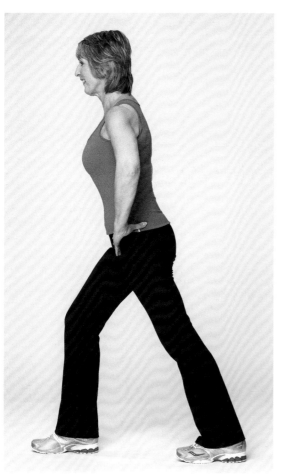
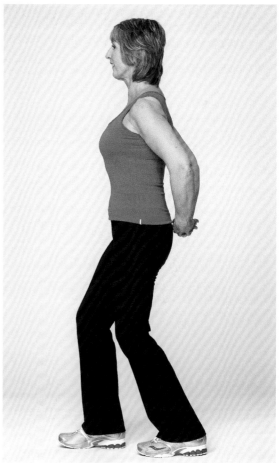

3 Front of hip stretch

Take your left leg behind you and stay on the ball of the foot. Now bend both knees and push the right hip further forwards to feel a stretch at the front of the right hip. Keep your body straight and directly above your hips. Hold for 10 seconds, then release. Change legs and repeat.

4 Front of thigh stretch

Stand tall and take hold of one ankle, using a chair or wall for support if necessary. Make sure your knees are in line with each other and that the standing leg is slightly bent. Hold for 10 seconds, then release. Change legs and repeat.

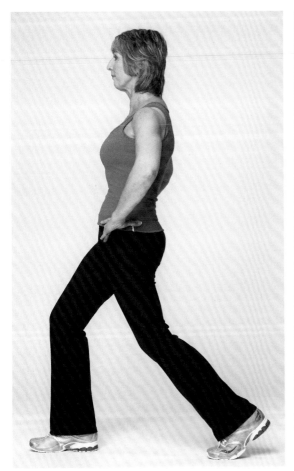 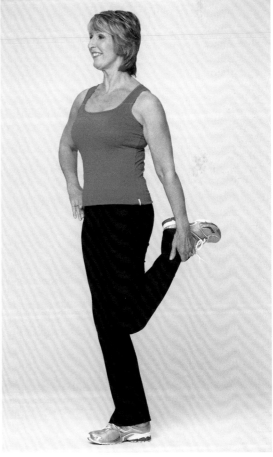

5 Inner thigh stretch

Stand with your legs wide and feet turned out slightly. Now bend your right leg, keeping your knee in line with the ankle, and turn the foot of the straight leg to face forwards, taking it far enough away from the right leg to feel a stretch in the inner thigh of the left leg. Hold for 10 seconds, then release. Change legs and repeat.

6 Back of thigh and hip stretch

Stand with one leg in front of the other and hip-width apart, with the front leg straight and the back leg bent. Lean forwards slightly, keeping your back straight and your head in line with your spine. Lift your hips up to feel a stretch in the back of the thigh and the hip of the back leg. Hold for 10 seconds, then release. Change legs and repeat.

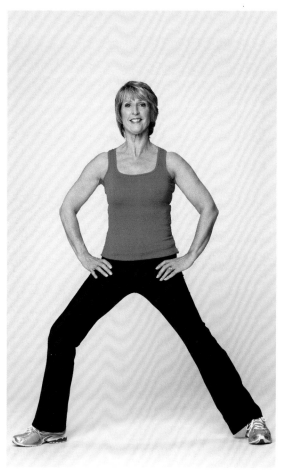

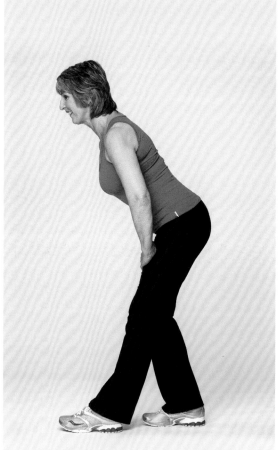

19
The Stay Young Hourglass Shape Workout

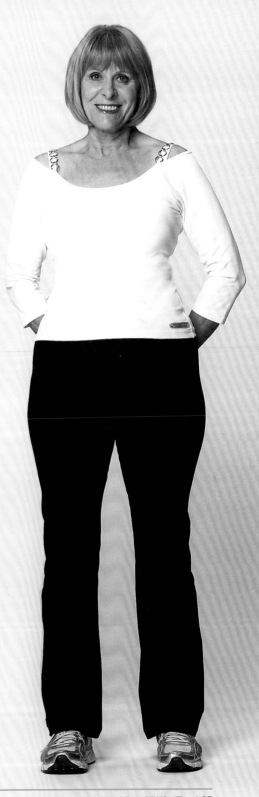

When we think of an hourglass figure we remember film stars such as Marilyn Monroe, Jane Mansfield and Diana Dors. They were beautiful women who had a voluptuous bosom, a small waist and shapely hips and they looked amazing. So, are *you* an hourglass shape?

If you have a largish bust and a visible waist, you will fall into this coveted category. You may feel your bust is too big, but if you lose weight your breasts will become smaller. In fact, everything will shrink.

My hourglass-shaped model is Maureen Hyndman, one of our franchisees for Rosemary Conley Diet & Fitness Clubs. Maureen operates her franchise in Rutland and East Leicestershire and, now in her 60s, is our oldest franchisee.

The best exercise for your body shape

To maintain your curves as you get older it's important for you to do plenty of aerobic activity to stay fit and healthy, but you also need an all-over toning programme to keep you looking shapely.

The aerobic schedule in the weekly exercise plan on page 188 will give you everything you need to keep trim and fit, while the toning workout will help you to maintain good muscle tone all over. If ever there was a body shape that was worth working on and maintaining, it's the hourglass figure!

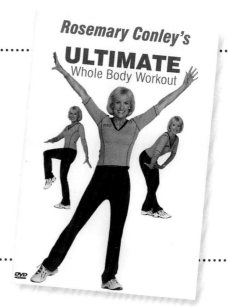

Recommended Rosemary Conley DVD:
Ultimate Whole Body Workout

This fitness DVD is perfect for an all-round exercise programme. It also includes a seated workout for anyone who finds it difficult to exercise standing up, so it's ideal for someone confined to a wheelchair or who has problems with balance.

The Hourglass Shape Toning Workout with weights

For your weights use ½ litre bottles of water or ½–1kg handweights. You will also need a sturdy chair.

Warm-up

Warm up for 5 minutes before you begin. March on the spot for 2 minutes Ⓐ. Roll your shoulders 10 times as you march. Then take 2 steps sideways, lifting your arms out to the sides as you step Ⓑ. Now do 8 side bends to alternate sides to warm up your waist Ⓒ, followed by 8 shallow squats to loosen your hips Ⓓ.

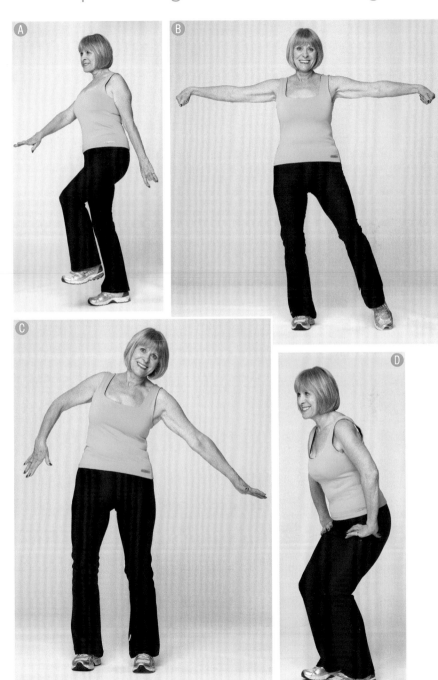

Toning programme

1 Leg and arm toning lunge with bicep curl

Start with one foot a large step ahead of the other and stay on the ball of the back foot. Hold a weight in each hand Ⓐ. Keep your weight centred between both legs and hold your tummy in tight. Now bend both knees and, at the same time, bring your hands up to meet your shoulders Ⓑ. Straighten your legs and arms and do a full set of reps before changing legs.

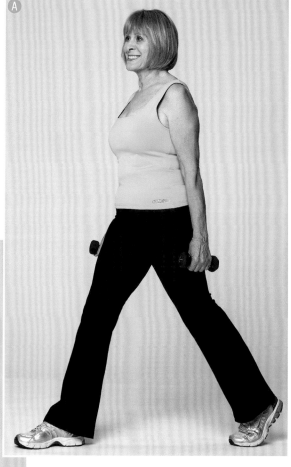

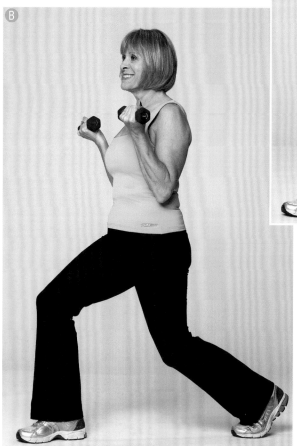

Beginners: Do 1 to 2 sets of 4 reps on each leg
Intermediate: Do 3 to 4 sets of 8 reps on each leg

2 Hip and thigh squat with arm raise

Stand with your feet hip-width apart and hold a handweight in each hand. Bend your knees, pushing your hips back and keeping your knees in line with your feet (A). As you lift up, bring one leg out to the side, with toes pointing forwards, and lift your arms to shoulder height (B). Lower and then repeat to the other side.

Variation: Do only the lower-body (leg) action, holding on to a chair for support.

Beginners: Do 1 to 2 sets of 16 reps (8 with each leg)
Intermediate: Do 3 to 4 sets of 20 reps (10 with each leg)

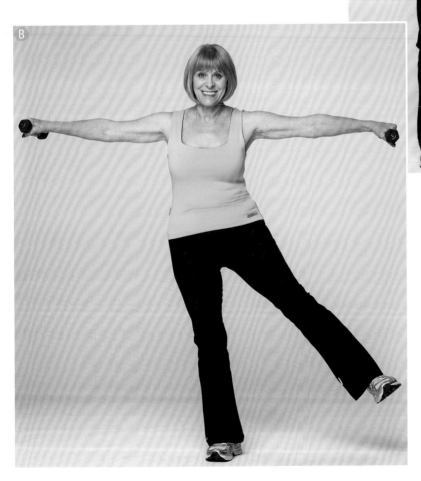

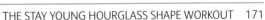

3 Shoulder shaper with leg strengthener

Stand with your feet just wider than shoulder-width apart and hold a handweight in each hand, with hands close together and the backs of your hands facing forwards Ⓐ. Lift both hands so that your elbows are higher than your wrists and, at the same time, bend your knees Ⓑ. Keep your body upright and your knees open in line with your feet and keep your shoulders down as the arms lift.

Beginners: Do 1 to 2 sets of 8 reps
Intermediate: Do 3 to 4 sets of 10 reps

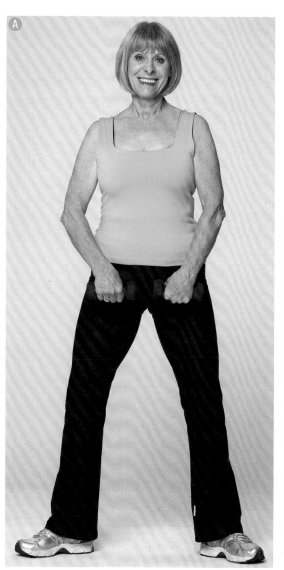

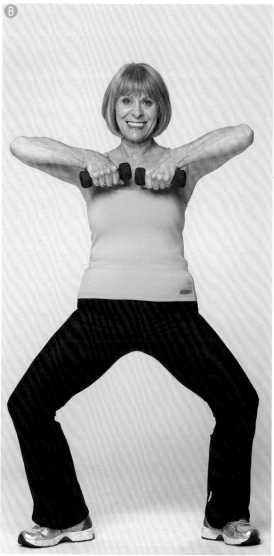

4 Underarm toner

Place the heels of your hands on the edge of the seat of a sturdy chair, with your feet flat on the floor and legs bent at a right angle Ⓐ. Now bend your elbows and lower your hips but keep your spine close to the chair seat Ⓑ. Push up again without locking your elbows, then repeat. Breathe in to lower and breathe out to lift.

Beginners:
Do 1 to 2 sets of 8 reps
Intermediate:
Do 3 to 4 sets of 10 reps

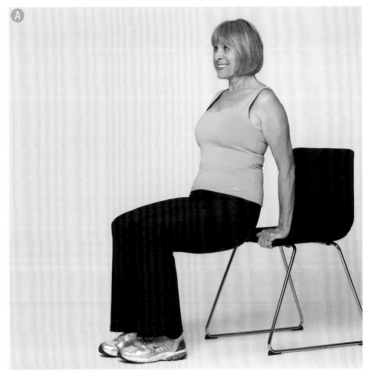

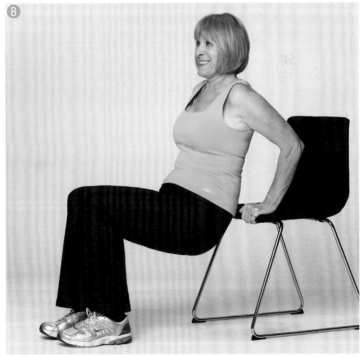

5 Bottom toner

Lie on your back with your lower calves up on the chair seat and your arms by your sides Ⓐ. Now, without arching your back, lift your hips off the floor Ⓑ, then lower them again. Breathe out as you lift and in as you lower and keep your neck and shoulders relaxed.

Beginners: Do 1 to 2 sets of 8 reps
Intermediate: Do 3 to 4 sets of 10 reps

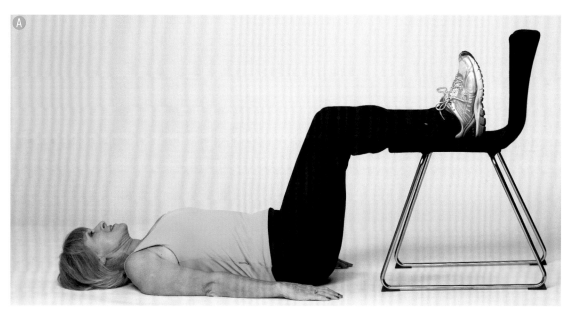

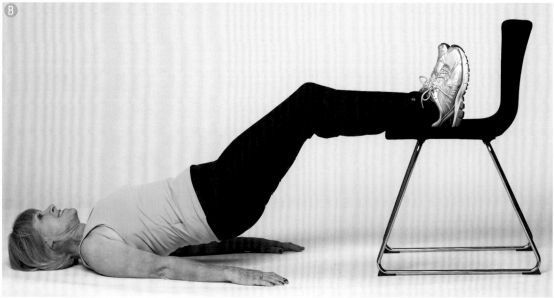

6 Tummy-flattening abdominal curl

Lie on your back with your lower calves up on the chair seat and your hands behind your head Ⓐ. Pull your tummy in and then lift your head and shoulders off the floor, keeping your chin off your chest Ⓑ. Lower again under control. Breathe out as you come up and breathe in as you lower.

Beginners: Do 1 to 2 sets of 8 reps
Intermediate: Do 3 to 4 sets of 10 reps

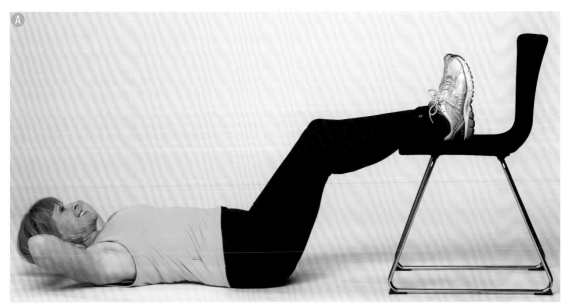

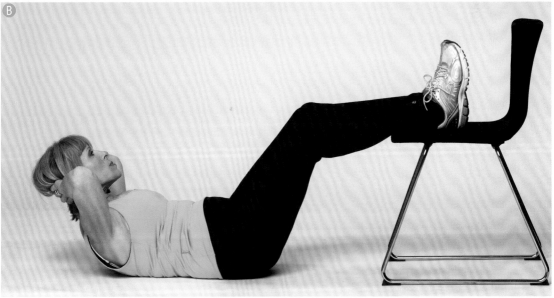

7 Waist-tightening curves

Lie on your back with your lower calves up on the chair seat and your hands behind your head Ⓐ. Pull your tummy in and lift your head and shoulders off the floor, keeping your chin off your chest, then reach round towards the chair leg on the right side with your right hand Ⓑ. Return to the centre and lower again, then lift and reach to the other side. Breathe out as you lift and curve, and breathe in as you straighten and lower.

Beginners: Do 1 to 2 sets of 8 reps
Intermediate: Do 3 to 4 sets of 10 reps

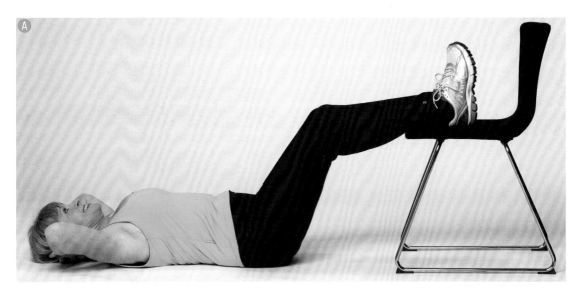

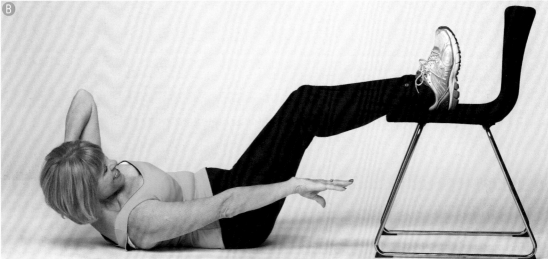

Now turn to page 185 to do the post-workout stretches.

The Hourglass Shape Toning Workout with resistance band

Warm-up

Warm up for 5 minutes before you begin. March on the spot for 2 minutes Ⓐ. Roll your shoulders 10 times as you march. Then do 8 small squats with feet apart Ⓑ, followed by 8 side bends to alternate sides with feet apart Ⓒ.

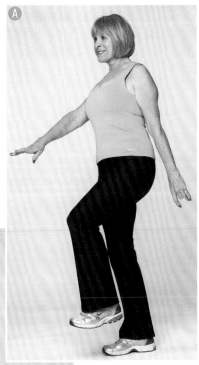

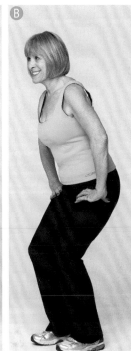

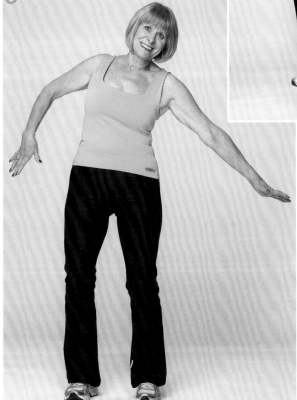

Toning programme

1 Thigh and bottom toner with underarm tightener

Stand with feet parallel and slightly wider than your hips. Holding the ends of the band in each hand, position the band across your hips, with your hands close to your hips and your elbows pointing back. Lean forwards slightly and pull your tummy in Ⓐ. Bend your knees in line with your feet and push your hips back as you straighten your elbows behind you Ⓑ. Then bend your elbows again and straighten your legs to return to the start position.

Beginners: Do 1 to 2 sets of 8 reps
Intermediate: Do 3 to 4 sets of 10 reps

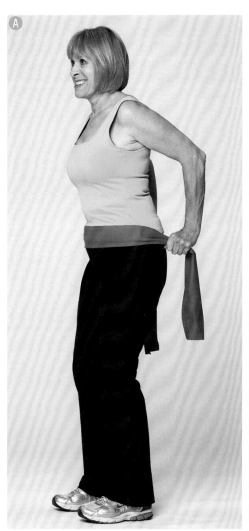
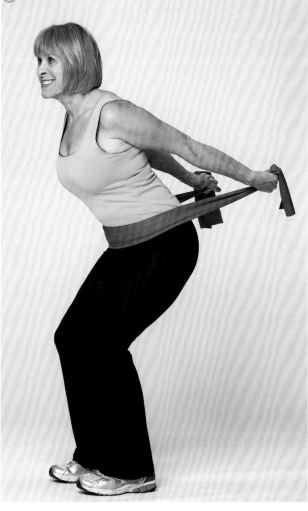

2 Bottom-toning hip raise

Lie on your back with knees bent, feet flat on the floor and hip-width apart. Place the band across your hips and secure it on the floor with your hands Ⓐ. Now lift your hips off the floor against the resistance of the band, without arching your back Ⓑ. Lower again, under control. Breathe out as you lift and in as you lower.

Beginners: Do 1 to 2 sets of 8 reps
Intermediate: See advanced exercise overleaf

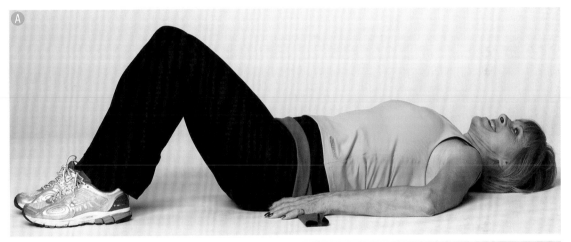

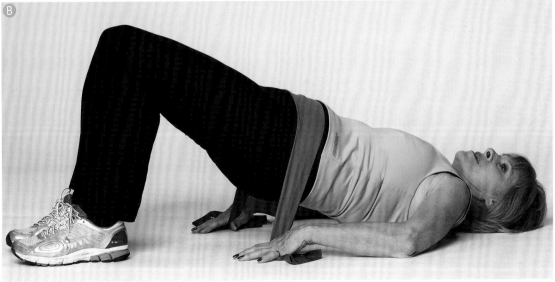

3 Advanced bottom toner

Lie on your back with your legs bent. Place the band across your hips and secure it on the floor with your hands. Bring your left ankle on top of your right knee Ⓐ. Now lift your hips off the floor without arching your back but keep the band firmly on the floor Ⓑ. Lower again, then lift and lower for a full set of reps before changing legs. Breathe out as you lift and in as you lower.

Intermediate only: Do 3 to 4 sets of 10 reps on each side

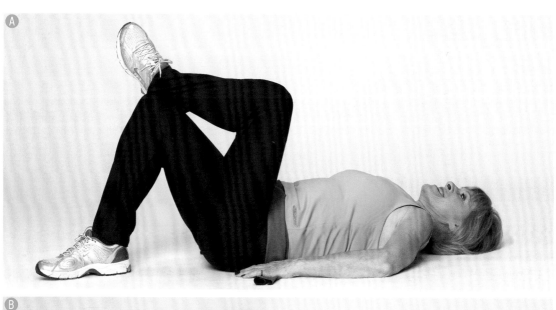

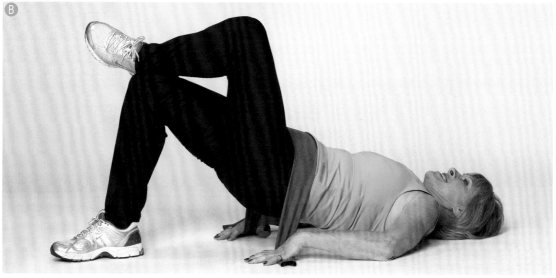

4 Waist-trimming twist

Lie on your back with the band placed under your shoulder blades and armpits and your left hand behind your head, holding the ends of the band in each hand Ⓐ. Now pull your tummy in tight, lift your head and shoulders off the floor and reach your right hand across to the left knee Ⓑ. Breathe in before you start and breathe out as you lift up and across. Keep repeating to the same side for a full set of reps and then change sides.

Beginners: Do 2 sets of 8 reps to each side
Intermediate: Do 4 sets of 8 reps to each side

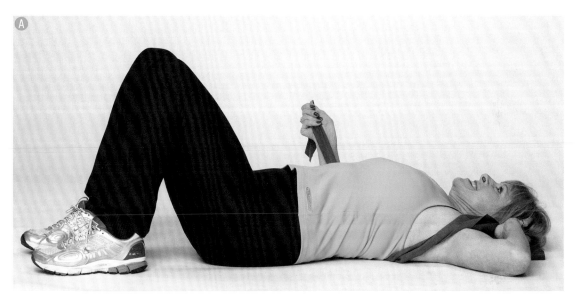

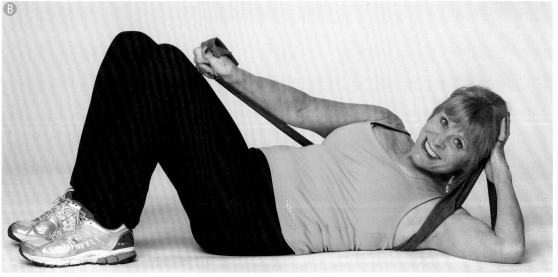

5 Tummy toner and bust shaper

Lie on your back with your knees bent and the band placed under your shoulder blades and armpits. Grip the band between your thumb and forefinger Ⓐ. Now, as you curl your upper body off the floor, extend your arms towards your knees Ⓑ, then lower again. Pull your tummy in tight and breathe out as you lift and in as you lower.

Beginners: Do 1 to 2 sets of 8 reps
Intermediate: Do 3 to 4 sets of 10 reps

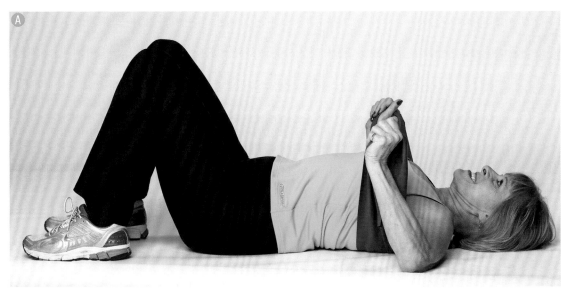

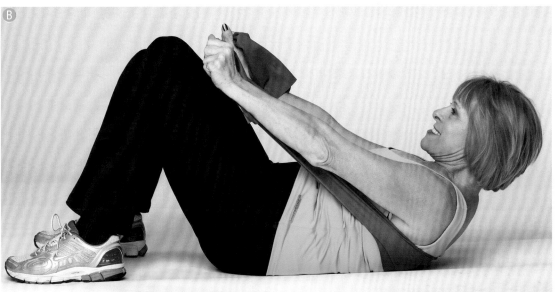

6 Outer thigh shaper

Wrap the band across your thighs, just above your knees, crossing it over underneath your thighs and bringing the ends on top of your legs. Hold the ends of the band in one hand, then lie on your side with your legs straight and in line with your body (if you prefer you can bend the bottom leg slightly to help you balance), and your toes pulling towards you. Support yourself with your free hand Ⓐ. Now lift the top leg to just above hip height and then lower it again, keeping your hips on top of each other and the leg straight and in line with the hip, with the heel pushing away from you Ⓑ so you feel the resistance of the band. Don't have the band too tight or it will restrict the movement of the top leg. Lift and lower the leg for a full set of reps before changing sides.

Beginners: Do 1 to 2 sets of 8 reps on each leg
Intermediate: Do 3 to 4 sets of 10 reps on each leg

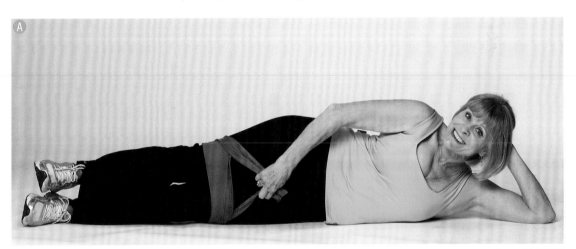

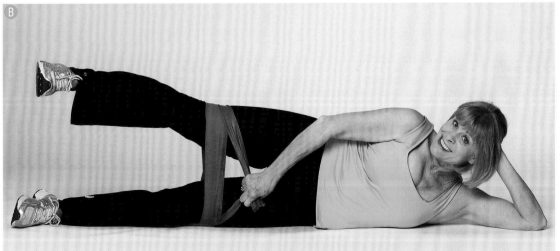

7 Spine strengthener and upper back toner

Lie on your front with the band placed across your upper back and secured on the floor with both hands, your legs outstretched and together and your forehead resting on the floor Ⓐ. Pull your tummy in, lift your head off the floor and push your arms out to the sides in line with your shoulders and clear of the floor if you can Ⓑ. Face the floor at all times. Hold for 2 seconds, then release.

Beginners: Do only 1 set of 6 reps
Intermediate: Do 2 sets of 6 reps

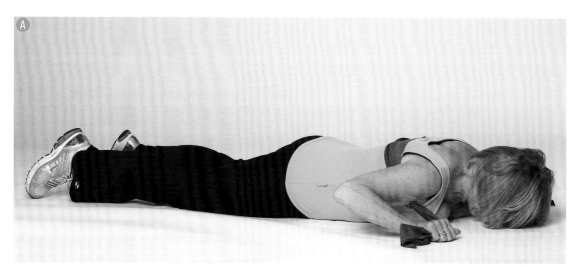

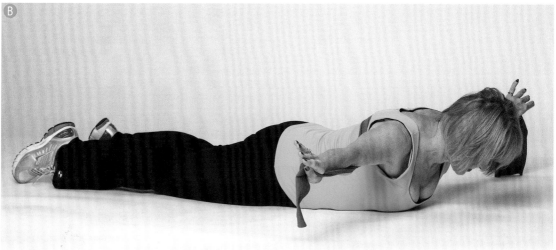

Now do the stretches below.

Post-Workout Stretches

1 Tricep stretch
Sit upright with your legs crossed and place one hand behind your shoulder. Use the other hand to gently press on the underarm and try to push the arm further down your back. Keep your head up and in line with your spine. Hold for 10 seconds, then release. Change arms and repeat.

2 Chest stretch
Bring both arms behind you on the floor. Sit upright and bring your shoulder blades together behind you to feel a stretch in your chest muscles. Hold for 10 seconds, then release.

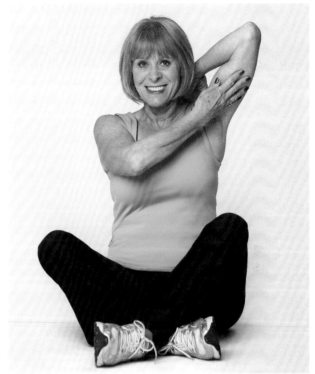

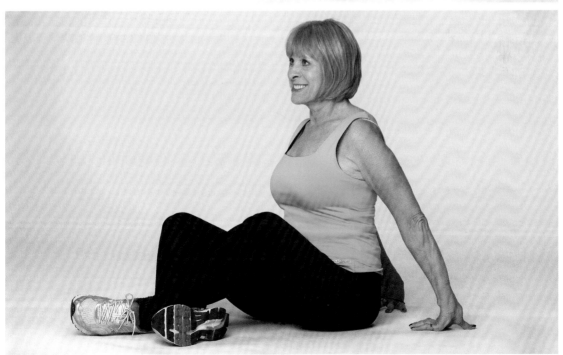

3 Outer thigh, waist and hip stretch

Extend both legs out in front, then bring your left foot over your right knee. Support your left knee with your right hand. Now lift your body upright and pull your left knee further across your body to feel a stretch in the left outer thigh and hip. Now look over your left shoulder, turning your shoulders slightly to the left to feel a stretch in the waist. Hold for 10 seconds, then release. Change legs and repeat.

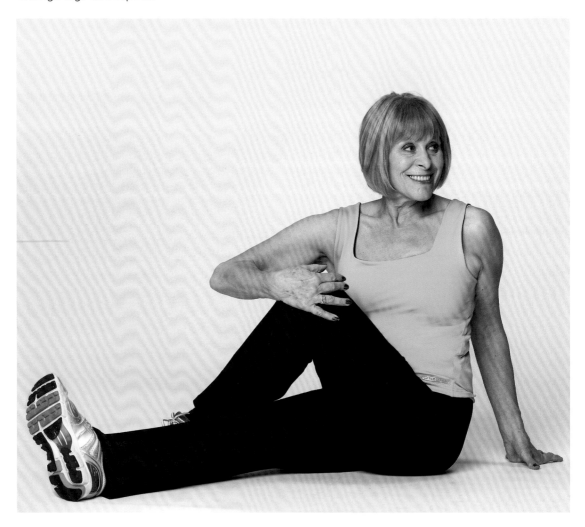

4 Front of thigh stretch

Lie on your front, bend one knee and hold it with the same-side hand. Rest your head on the other hand and relax your upper body. Now bring your knees together, pressing the hip of the bent leg into the floor. Hold for 10 seconds, then release. Repeat with the other leg.

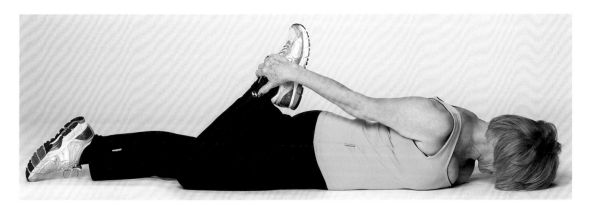

5 Tummy stretch

Still lying on your front, place your bent forearms out to the sides, with your elbows under your shoulders. Now lift your head and shoulders off the floor and support yourself on your elbows, lifting your chin slightly to feel a stretch down the abdominal area. Hold for 10 seconds, then release.

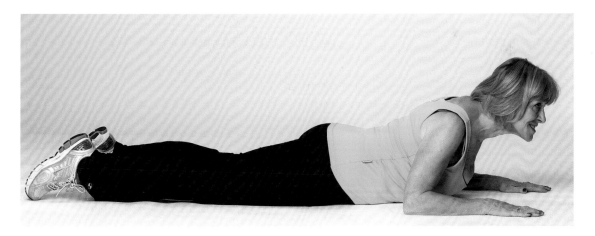

Hourglass Shape Weekly Exercise Plan

Day	Type	Beginners	Intermediate
1	Cardio	Walk or cycle 20 mins	Power walk 30 mins
2	Hourglass Shape Toning Workout		
3	Cardio/tone	Do DVD whole programme or an aerobics class OR Power walk 20 mins + Hourglass Shape Toning Workout	Do DVD whole programme or an aerobics class OR Row, cycle or cross-trainer 30 mins + Hourglass Shape Toning Workout
4	Cardio	Walk or swim 20 mins	Power walk or swim 40 mins +
5	Hourglass Shape Toning Workout		Hourglass Shape Toning Workout
6	Cardio/tone	Walk, cycle or swim 20 mins + Hourglass Shape Toning Workout	Power walk on a route with some incline 40 mins + Hourglass Shape Toning Workout
7	Cardio/tone	Do DVD whole programme OR Power walk 25 mins + Hourglass Shape Toning Workout	Do DVD whole programme OR Row, cycle or cross-trainer 30 mins + Hourglass Shape Toning Workout

MONITOR YOUR PROGRESS

	Weight	BMI	Waist-to-hip ratio
Start			
End month 1			
End month 2			
End month 3			
End month 4			

Post-Cardio Stretches

Learn these stretches so that they can be done after every aerobic activity. They will help to keep your muscles extended and prevent aching later.

1 Calf stretch
Stand with one foot in front of the other, with both feet pointing forwards and the back foot as far back as possible. Bend the front knee in line with the ankle to feel a strong stretch in the calf of the back leg. Hold for 10 seconds, then release. Change legs and repeat.

2 Lower calf and chest stretch
Stand upright with one foot slightly ahead of the other, feet hip-width apart and both knees bent to feel a stretch in the lower calf. At the same time, take both hands behind you and open your shoulders to feel a stretch across your chest. Hold for 10 seconds, then release. Change sides and repeat.

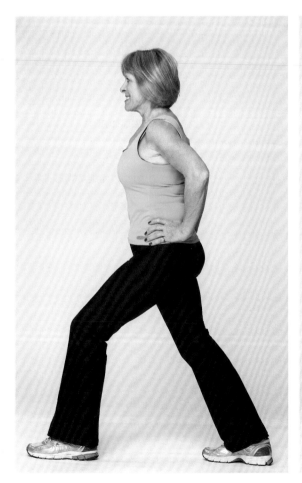

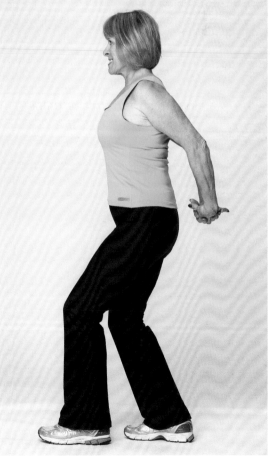

3 Front of hip stretch

Take your left leg behind you and stay on the ball of that foot. Now bend both knees and push your left hip further forwards to feel a stretch at the front of that hip. Keep your body straight and directly above your hips. Hold for 10 seconds, then release. Change legs and repeat.

4 Front of thigh stretch

Stand tall and take hold of one ankle, using a chair or wall for support if necessary. Make sure that your knees are in line with each other and the standing leg is slightly bent. Hold for 10 seconds, then release. Change legs and repeat.

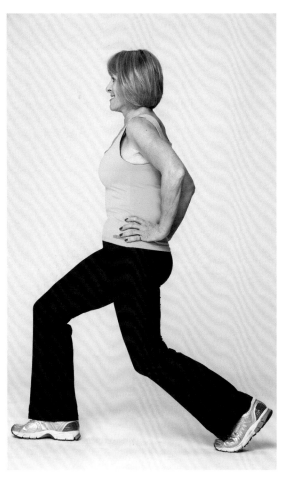

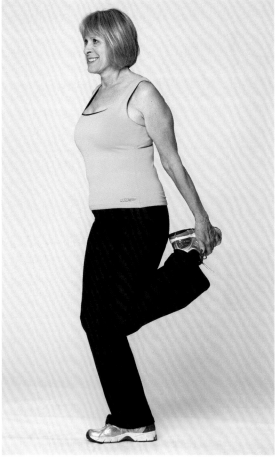

5 Inner thigh stretch

Stand with your legs wide and your feet turned out slightly. Now bend your right leg, keeping the knee in line with the ankle and, at the same time, turn the foot of the straight leg to point forwards and take it far enough away from your right leg to feel a stretch in the inner thigh of the left leg. Hold for 10 seconds, then release. Repeat to the other side.

6 Back of thigh and hip stretch

Stand with one leg in front of the other and feet hip-width apart, with your front leg straight and your back leg bent. Lean forwards slightly, keeping your back straight and your head in line with your spine. Lift your hips to feel a stretch in the back of the thigh and the hip of the front leg. Hold for 10 seconds, then release. Change legs and repeat.

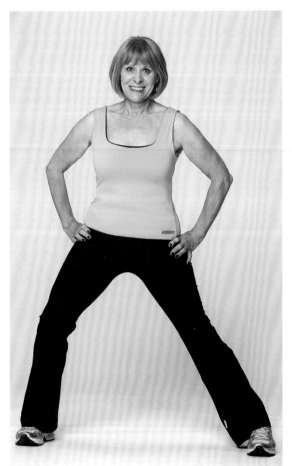

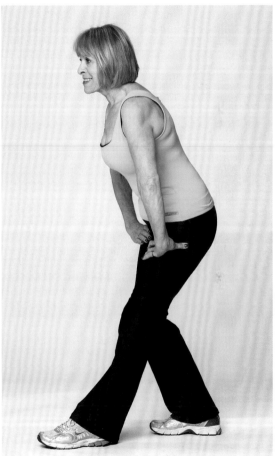

20
The Forever Young Workout

When a trial was undertaken to see how quickly older people increased their fitness through regular exercise compared to younger folk, the results were amazing. It turned out that age made no difference. Whether the volunteers were in their 20s or their 80s, regular exercise increased their fitness at a similar rate.

As we get older exercise is even more crucial to our health. If we are to live to reach our 100th birthday – and it is reported that 11 million of us alive today will do just that – we need to enjoy good health on the journey to that milestone. But there's no point in living that long if we're immobile or bedridden. We want to be fit and able, fun to be with and happy in ourselves, and we *can* be if we have a positive attitude, eat healthily, stay active and keep our bodies moving.

Exercise is one of the most important factors in keeping our muscles and bones strong. If we have strong muscles and bones we're less likely to 'shrink' as so many older folk do. Our sense of balance will be better, our motor skills will be maintained and our flexibility can remain youthful. Exercise helps the brain to stay youthful too. There really is no downside to taking regular exercise.

Two people in their 80s who particularly inspire me are the Queen and my mother-in-law, Jeanne. Her Majesty Queen Elizabeth II is 85 years young as I write this book and looks amazing – fit and alert and totally able to fulfil her incredible duties as our monarch. Her Majesty has been physically active all her life – by horse riding, dancing and walking, amongst other activities. Such activities have stood her in good stead as she has reached her later years.

My mother-in-law, Jeanne, is 89 years young and is remarkable. Totally mentally alert and with better eyesight than mine, Jeanne needs no hearing aid and no walking stick. She can walk up the 38 stairs to her flat in our house without stopping and breathes quite normally when she gets there.

Jeanne used to be a yoga teacher in her earlier years and kept practising her yoga exercises until a couple of years ago when she became quite poorly. She was living on her own then as her husband had passed away some nine years previously and up to that time she had looked after herself at their family home. It was then, after a short stay in hospital, that it was decided that Jeanne should move in with us.

Jeanne is a joy to have around. A whizz with the sewing machine and able to do any hand-sewing that we need, she occupies herself reading the newspapers, doing crosswords and watching the Test Match on television (she loves her cricket!). Jeanne also makes all her own birthday, Christmas and Easter cards and has recently written her autobiography. For years she made all her own clothes but now she enjoys wearing some of mine and just lengthens the skirts by adding a panel of fabric above the waist, which allows the original fabric of the skirt to drop down and the skirt to appear much longer.

About 18 months ago, Jeanne had a fall at the dentist's. She missed the bottom step of the stairs and twisted her ankle badly. It was very painful and it took several weeks for it to get back to normal.

Initially Jeanne couldn't walk on it at all and we wheeled her about her flat in an office chair that had castors, before investing in a wheelchair that was easier to manoeuvre. Jeanne has always managed to bathe herself, but with such a painful ankle, getting out of the bath proved extremely difficult, even with my helping to support her. Getting in wasn't too bad, it was the getting out that was trickier, but we seemed to manage – until two weeks into the recovery.

Suddenly, Jeanne couldn't find enough strength in her legs to lift herself up from the base of the bath. As I straddled the bath, which was now empty of water, I managed to lift her up and help her out of the bath but it was a real struggle.

Then it dawned on me. After just two weeks of not walking up and down those 38 stairs to her flat, Jeanne had lost muscle strength in her legs. Having initially thought we needed to get her a physiotherapist, I worked it out that if she could just exercise by standing up and sitting down from a chair repetitively, she would be strengthening her front thigh muscles, which had not been adequately used since her accident.

I asked Jeanne to do 10 stand-up-sit-downs four times a day every day to see if we could strengthen her legs again. Very willingly and with total dedication she did just that and, within a week, she had regained her strength in her legs and was able to lift herself out of the bath again! By week five we didn't need the wheelchair and Jeanne was well on the road to full recovery.

This whole experience really made me think. I then devised a workout using a resistance band to strengthen other parts of Jeanne's body. Being fitter and stronger gave Jeanne added confidence, which has stood her in good stead in her everyday life.

Here is the workout I created for her and I hope it will work for you or your older loved ones. It only takes a few minutes and, if you practise these exercises three times a week, it will make a real difference in helping you to maintain your muscle strength and keep your bones strong.

The Forever Young Workout

All of these exercises are done from a sturdy dining chair.

Warm-Up

1 Ankle circles

Sit on the front half of a sturdy dining chair and circle one ankle 5 times in one direction and then 5 times in the opposite direction. Repeat with the other foot.

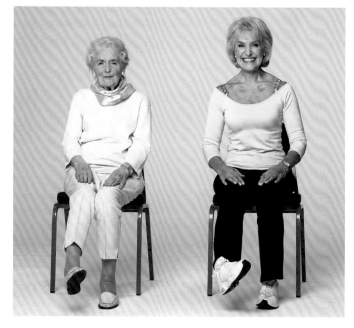

2 Wrist circles

Sitting upright, circle both hands from the wrist in an outwards direction 8 times, then repeat in an inwards direction.

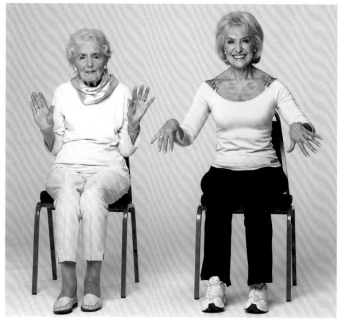

3 Sitting march

Sitting securely on the front half of the chair, do 20 marching steps on the spot, allowing your bent arms to swing at your sides as you march. Try to hold your tummy in throughout, but breathe normally.

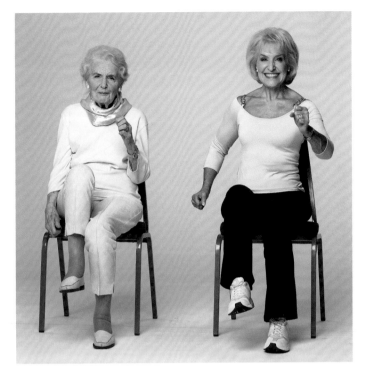

4 Sitting side bends

Sitting upright and securely on the front half of the chair, slowly curve your body to one side and allow the hand on that side to lower with you. Come up to the centre and then repeat to the other side with the other hand lowering towards the floor. Keep the movement slow and rhythmical. Do 8 in total, alternating sides (4 to each side).

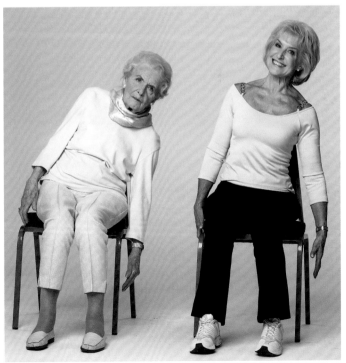

5 Leg lifts

Sitting upright and securely on the front half of the chair, hold on to the chair seat with your hands. Now straighten one leg out in front, but keep both thighs in line with each other. Lower the leg again and repeat with the other leg. Do 6 with each leg, alternating legs (12 in total).

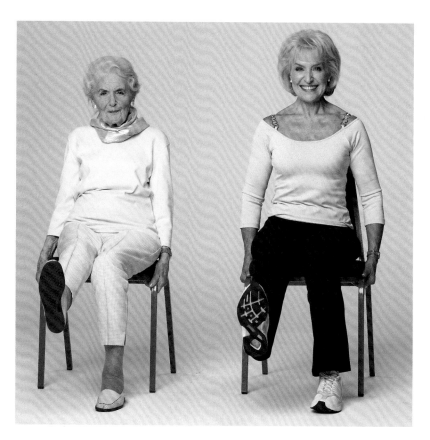

You are now ready to start your **Resistance Band Workout**.

The Forever Young Resistance Band Workout

These exercises will really help you to maintain your muscle strength and keep your bones strong into your mature years.

> **Tips on using the resistance band**
> - Always hold the band between your thumbs and index fingers.
> - Do not wrap the band around your hands at any time as this can stop the blood circulation.
> - Before you begin each exercise, keep the band taut, not loose, for greatest benefit.

1 Posture improver

Sitting securely on the front half of the chair, take the band and place it across your open hands, palms facing upwards, as if holding a tray. Keeping the band taut and your elbows fixed to your waist Ⓐ, pull the band wider Ⓑ, then relax it. Feel this exercise working the muscles in your upper back and shoulders to improve your posture.

Do 6 times, then rest and repeat if possible. To make the exercise harder, make the band shorter at the start of the exercise.

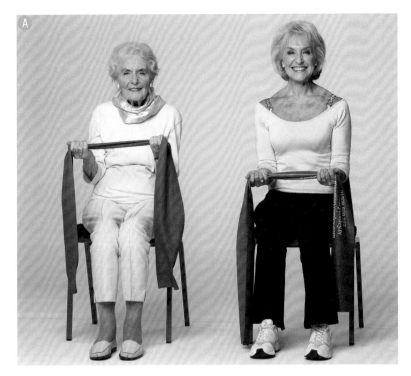

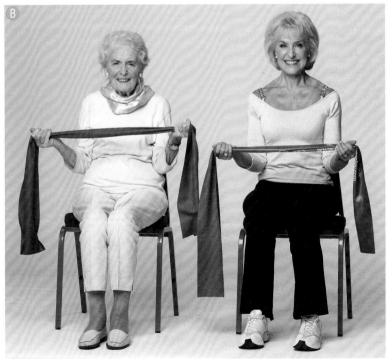

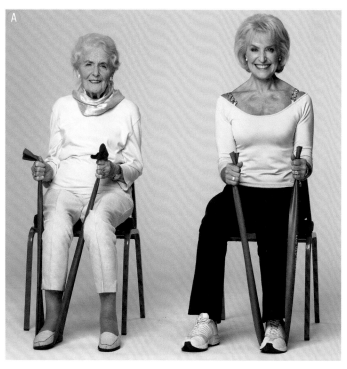

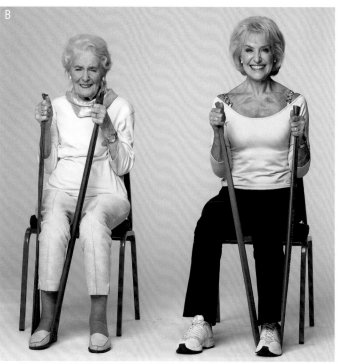

2 Wrist and arm strengthener

Place the band underneath one foot and take hold of each end with your hands Ⓐ. Rest the heel of that foot firmly on the floor. Keeping your elbows touching your waist, bend your arms and bring your hands closer to your shoulders Ⓑ. Slowly lower them again, then keep lifting and lowering.

Do 6 times in total, then rest and repeat if you can. This exercise strengthens the front of your arms and your wrists.

3 Shoulder strengthener ▶

Sitting upright on the front half of the chair and holding your tummy in, place one end of the band under one foot to secure it. Hold the other end in your hand and out at the side Ⓐ. Extend the band to shoulder height if possible Ⓑ, then lower it again. Keep the movement smooth and controlled.

Do 6 reps, then change legs, securing the band under the other foot, and repeat. Repeat one more set of 6 reps on each side if possible. This exercise helps to keep your arms and shoulders strong and improves your posture.

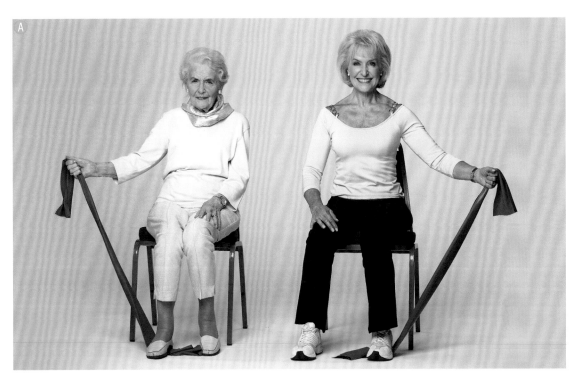

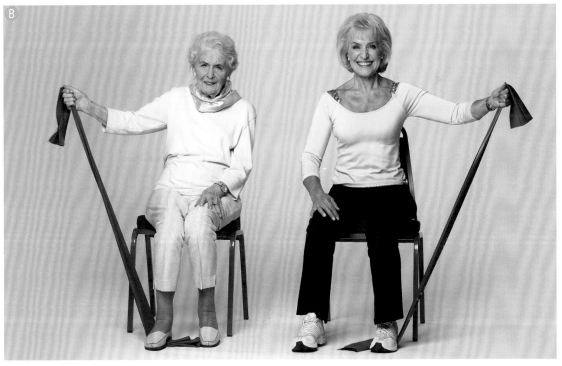

4 Chest toner

Place the band around your back and hold one end in each hand as it comes around the body under the armpits. The band should be taut and your arms bent Ⓐ. Now straighten your arms out in front at shoulder height, keeping your shoulders down Ⓑ. Bend your arms again and repeat.

Do 8 reps, then rest and repeat. This works the muscles in your chest.

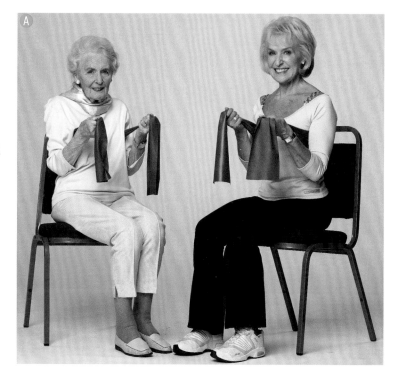

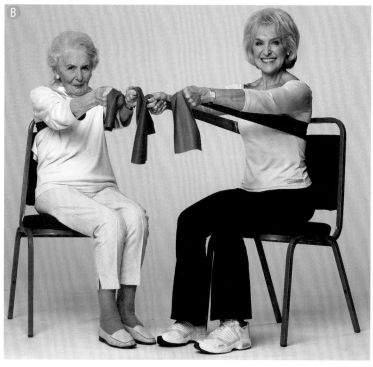

5 Outer thigh and hip strengthener

Sit in the front half of the chair seat with knees together and feet shoulder-width apart. Wrap the band over and then under the lower part of your thighs, securing the ends in your hands, and rest your hands on top of your thighs Ⓐ. Keeping a firm hold of the band, pull your knees apart in line with your feet Ⓑ. Release your knees again and then pull out and in again 10 times in total.

Rest and repeat another set. This will keep your hips really strong.

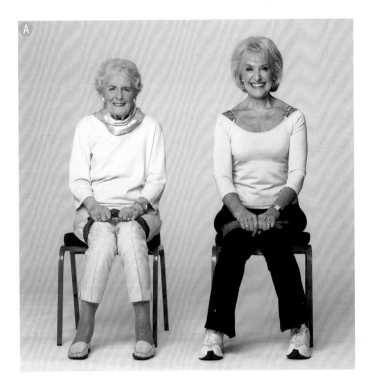

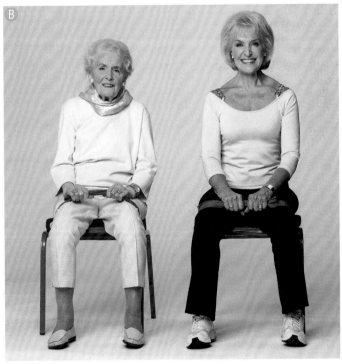

6 Stand up sit down

Sit on the front half of the chair seat with your feet flat on the floor and then take them back a little further. Place your hands on top of your thighs or on the sides of the chair seat to help you push Ⓐ, and lean forwards. Now stand up fairly swiftly in one movement Ⓑ and then sit down very slowly, taking 3–4 seconds if you can Ⓒ.

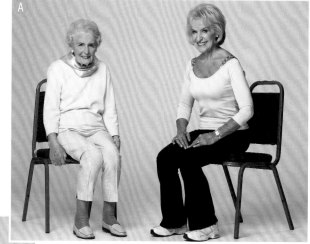

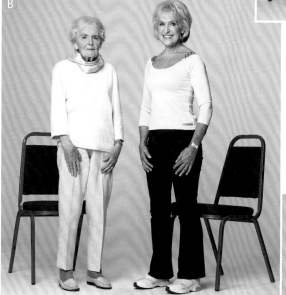

Do up to 10 reps. This exercise strengthens the large leg muscles.

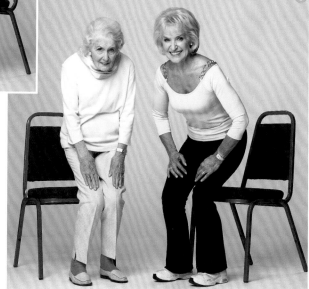

7 Hand wringing

Roll up the band into a tight roll (this is a very good finger exercise) and hold the ends in your hands. Now imagine wringing out clothes as you twist the roll of band in one direction and back again to strengthen your wrists.

Do 6 reps, then repeat, reversing the direction.

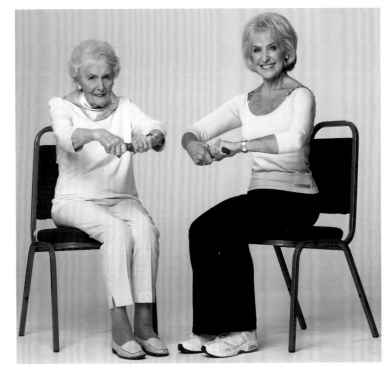

Stretches

To help relax your muscles do the following stretches at the end of your workout.

1 Shoulder stretch

Sit securely on your sturdy dining chair and extend your hands in front of your shoulders, dropping your head slightly to stretch out the shoulder area. Hold for 6 seconds, then release.

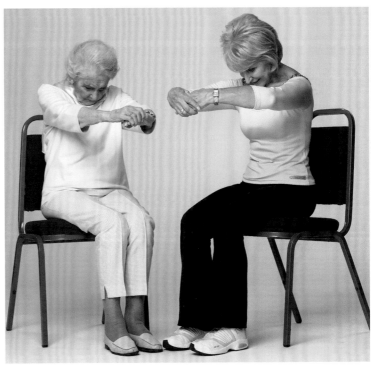

2 Chest stretch

Sitting securely on the front half of the chair, place your hands behind you on the edges of the back of the chair. Lean forwards slightly to feel a stretch across your chest. Hold for 6 seconds, then release.

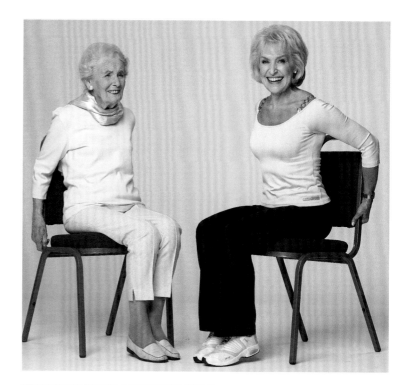

3 Back of leg stretch

Sitting securely on the front half of the chair, keep one leg bent with the foot flat on the floor and extend the other leg straight out in front of you and rest the heel on the floor. Place your hands on the sides of the chair seat or on your thigh and lean forwards slightly to feel a stretch in the back of the knee and thigh of the straight leg. Hold for 6 seconds. Take a deep breath in and as you breathe out, lean forwards a little further to feel more of a stretch. Hold for a further 6 seconds. Change legs and repeat.

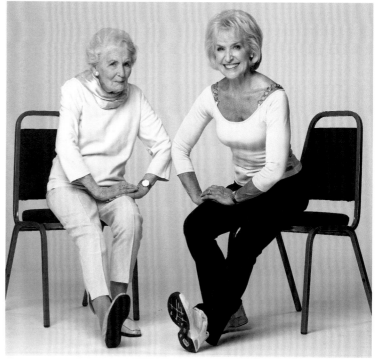

4 Front of thigh stretch

Stand up and hold on to the back of the chair with one hand. Using the chair for support, lift one leg, bend the knee and take hold of your ankle or trouser leg. Aim to keep the knees together. By bending the lower leg backwards you should feel a stretch down the front of the thigh. To feel more of a stretch, ease the hip forwards. Hold for 6 seconds, then change legs and repeat.

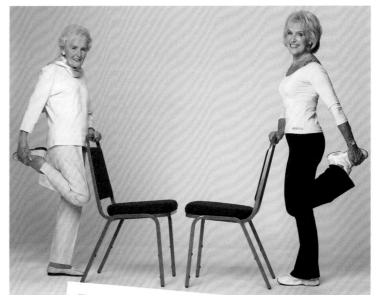

Postscript

On the day Jeanne came to our offices at Quorn House for the photo shoot for this book she didn't know what to expect. Nor did anyone else! Her ability to do everything we asked and her gentle grace and youthful attitude left everyone amazed and inspired.

At the end of the day Mike, my husband (and of course Jeanne's son), joined us for a family photo. It was a lovely way to end a very special day and too nice a photo not to include in this book.

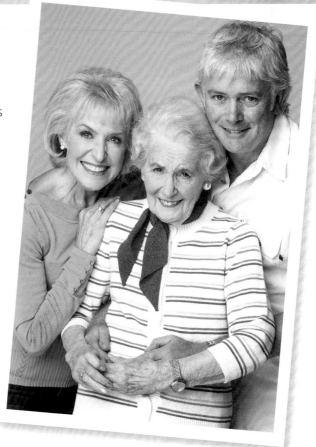

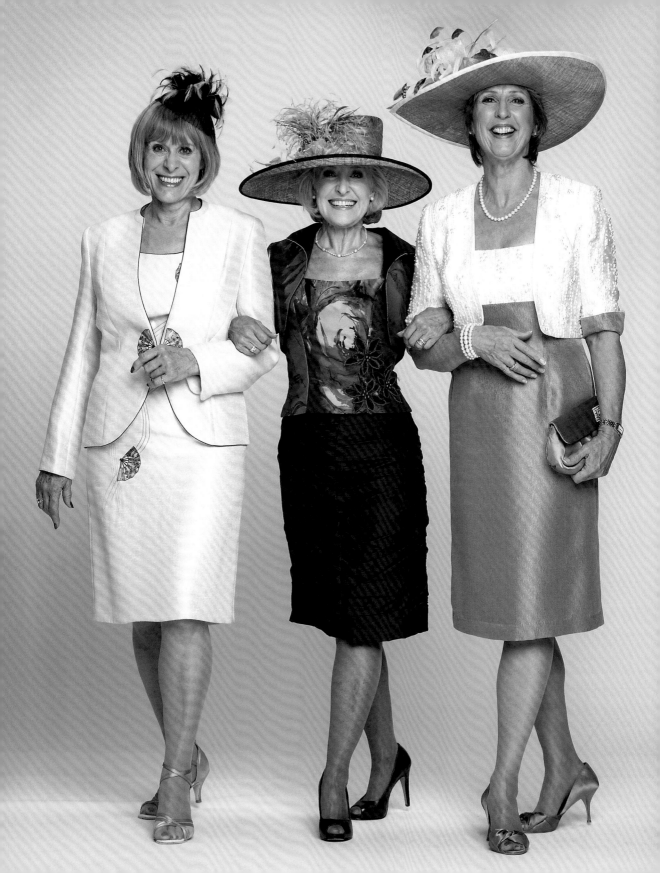

21
Dressing for your figure shape

As we mature, dressing appropriately and in a flattering style for our figure shape can make us look years younger. The correct skirt length, shaped jacket, neckline, sleeve length and, of course, colour can transform our look from dowdy to trendy without us ever looking like 'mutton dressed as lamb'.

The golden rule is to cover up any bits of your body that you know are showing the signs of ageing. There's nothing more of a giveaway of our age than to expose the bits of our bodies that look as if they could do with a good iron! A crinkly cleavage, wrinkly arms, varicose vein legs and a spare tyre around the middle all need covering up and we can do it subtly without it appearing obvious that's what we are doing.

It's a good idea also to 'test' what you are going to wear by moving around in front of a mirror – leaning forwards, sitting down, and so on. Make sure you look in a reverse mirror too and *always* use a full-length mirror.

For some great fashion advice take a look at my *Diet & Fitness* magazine and read celebrity stylist Nicky Hambleton-Jones's brilliant advice. She's a real expert in knowing what suits who and she gives some great guidance into the latest fashions. Check out her website www.nhjstyle.com for more information.

To illustrate this chapter I asked my friend and colleague Mary Morris (who is an apple shape) and our only franchisee aged over 60, Maureen Hyndman (an hourglass shape), to join me (a pear shape) for a photo shoot to illustrate our different styles of dressing to flatter our figure shapes. We all have daughters who got married in the last year or so, and in the picture opposite we are wearing our wedding outfits. Maureen (left) is an hourglass shape with a larger bust, a clear waistline and curvy hips and thighs. I (centre) am showing my bigger hips and thighs but narrower waist and smaller bust, typical of a pear shape. Mary (right) is an apple shape with slim hips and thighs but a wider waist.

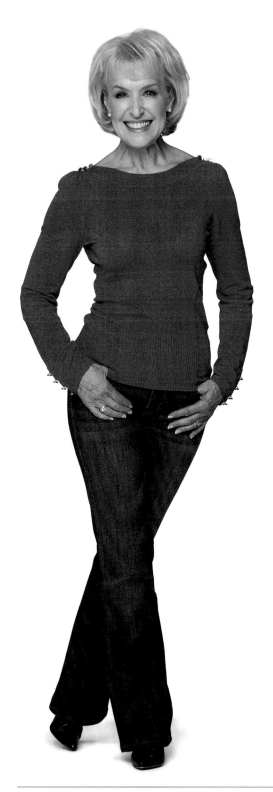

Pear shape – casual wear

The bootleg jeans balance my heavier thighs by having a wider leg at the bottom. The bright red top draws the eye above the hips, and the slim-fit styling around the middle shows off a pear-shape's best feature – the waist. The buttons on the shoulder add width, giving a better balance and proportion to a pear-shaped figure.

Pear shape – evening wear

This evening dress is made of stretch fabric so it shows my curves and is embroidered with white beads that add detail to the bust and the bottom of the skirt and divert attention away from my hips and thighs. The shoulders are the last part of a pear shape's arms to show the signs of ageing so they can go bare for longer but I'm wearing very long satin gloves to cover my arms, as arms are not the best feature on a pear shape.

Pear shape – wedding wear

This three-piece outfit comprises a ruched skirt in plain satin to play down the hips, a snugly fitting bodice and short, bolero-style jacket, both patterned, but drawing the eye upwards and accentuating a pear shape's slim waist.

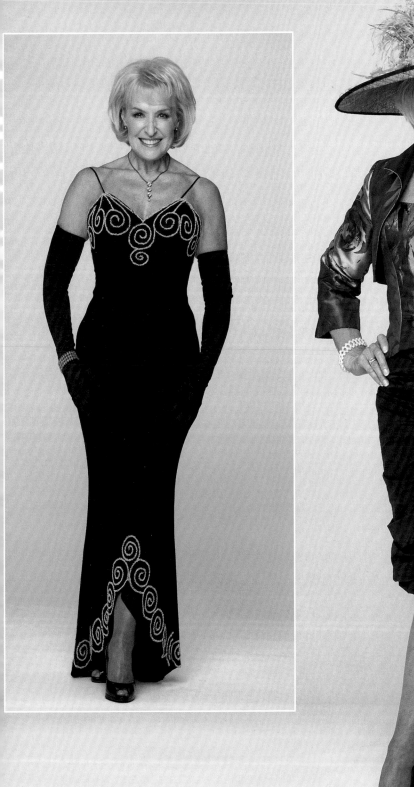
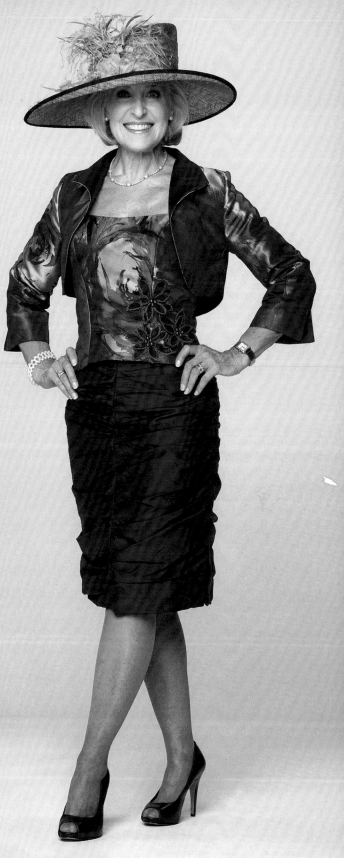

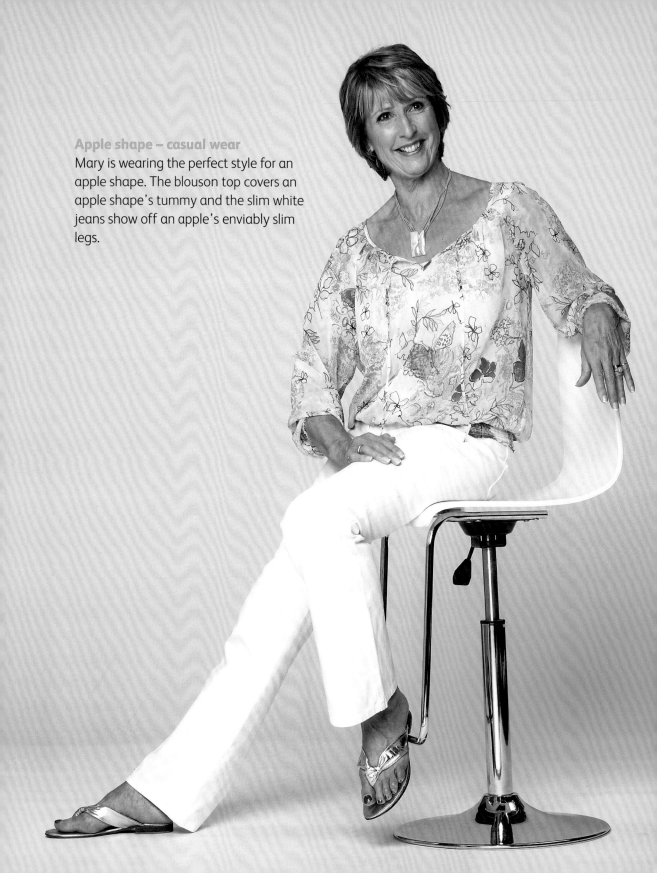

Apple shape – casual wear
Mary is wearing the perfect style for an apple shape. The blouson top covers an apple shape's tummy and the slim white jeans show off an apple's enviably slim legs.

Apple shape – evening wear

This beautifully cut evening dress has a low-cut neckline and clever styling to the side of the abdomen, with a diamante detail, to give the illusion of a smaller waist. As apple shapes keep their lovely arms looking youthful for longer, a sleeveless dress looks great on them.

Apple shape – wedding wear

Mary's exquisite wedding outfit is perfect for an apple shape. The pear-encrusted detail across the bust of the dress and in the short jacket draw the eye upwards and away from the abdominal area. The plain silk lower part of the dress is so beautifully styled it gives a wonderful waistline.

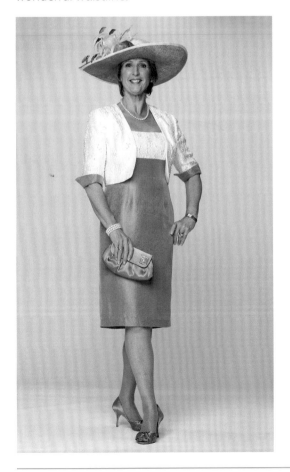

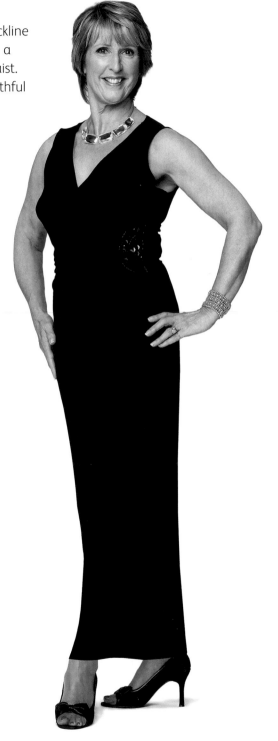

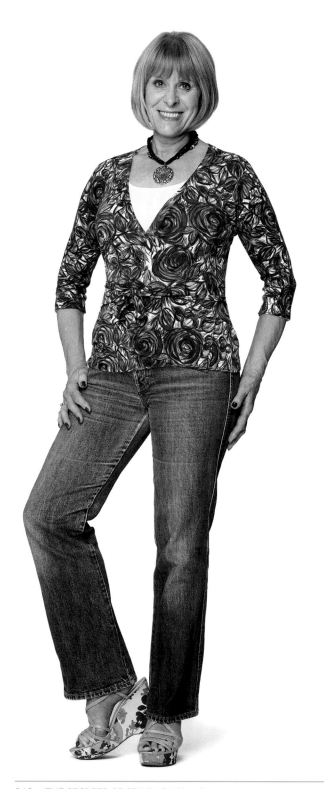

Hourglass shape – casual wear

Maureen is wearing straight-cut jeans and a three-quarter-length sleeved wrap-over top to accentuate her curves. Wearing a white 'body' underneath gives a younger, 'layered' look and covers the cleavage, which looks better concealed as you get older.

Hourglass shape – evening wear

Maureen's wonderfully bright evening dress suits her beautifully, with a carefully styled upper body to flatter her ample bust and wide-enough straps to cover the wider straps of a support bra. The fitted style shows off her waist and the floaty skirt skims over her hips. The chiffon stole can be used to cover the arms if needed and can also help keep you warm on a chilly evening.

Hourglass shape – wedding wear

Maureen's wedding suit is perfect for her shape as the detail on the jacket draws the eye in to the waist. An hourglass's slim ankles means that Maureen can get away with ankle straps as they are fine and crisscrossed downwards. However, an horglass shape should avoid straight-across ankle straps as they can have the effect of shortening the leg.

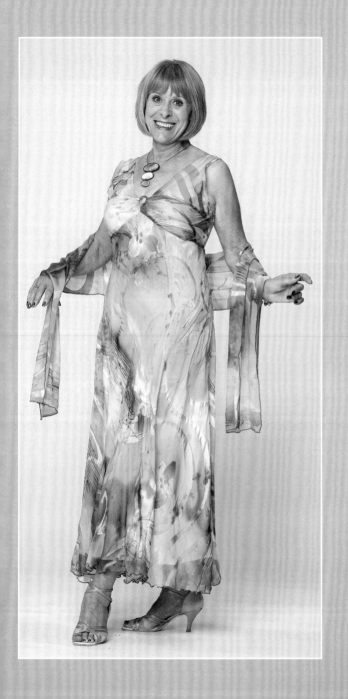
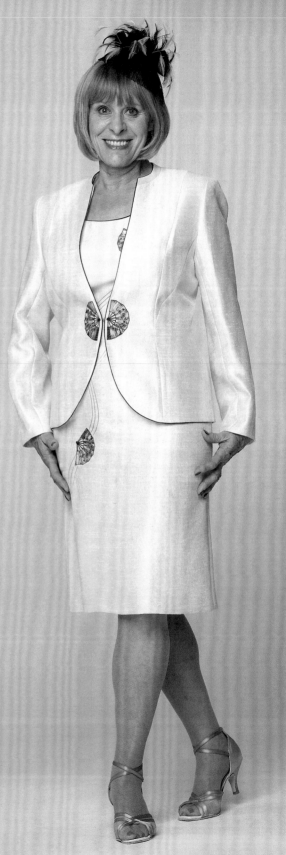

What are the best styles for your figure shape?

Here are my golden rules to help *you* dress to flatter *your* figure and your age.

Pear Shape

- **Small waist:** Wear styles that accentuate your waistline: short jackets, fitted styles with an A-line skirt, dresses with an empire line. If you're tall, you can wear belts to accentuate your slim waist, but shorter women may find this too cluttering.
- **Good ankles:** Wear skirts that show your slim ankles, and wear high heels if possible to add length to your legs. Avoid ankle straps as these will make your legs look fatter and shorter. Wear good-quality tights with Lycra. (I wear Pretty Polly Nylons in 'Highlight' colour. These aren't cheap but they transform my legs and, as they are just 10 denier, they look invisible. They are highly effective in making those pins look attractive.)
- **Small bust:** Make sure you wear a bra that maximises your bust. Wear lighter or brighter colours or patterns above the waist and don't be afraid to wear striking jewellery and the occasional frill or large collar.
- **Flattish stomach:** Show off your flatter stomach with an uncluttered waistline. Avoid anything gathered, elasticated or pleated.
- **Narrow shoulders:** Wear tops with shoulder detail such as frills or trims to widen the shoulders. Horizontal stripes above the waist work really well too.

Worst points

- **Wide hips:** Always wear plain or dark colours below the waist. Keep lines simple.
- **Large thighs:** A-line or straight skirts, not too long or too short, are most flattering. Bootleg-style jeans work wonders for pear shapes, while slim-fit and skinny-fit styles should be avoided. In the summer, wear only longer-length shorts for a more flattering look.
- **Large arms:** A pear shape's arms don't age well. Wear three-quarter or full-length sleeves for the most flattering look.

Apple Shape

Best points

- **Generous bust:** Always wear a correctly fitting bra to enhance your bustline. Blouson-style tops look great on apple shapes, as do 'bomber'-style jackets as they accentuate your slim hips and show off your legs.
- **Slim arms:** Your arms will look good into old age, so you'll look fab in sleeveless tops and dresses.

- **Slim hips and thighs:** You can wear high-waisted slimfit jeans and look stunning in them. You can also wear lighter colours and patterns below the waist. You'll look great in shorts and your legs will be the envy of any pear shape!

- **Thick waist and abdomen:** Wear styles such as bright or patterned jackets that cover your waist and abdomen but show off your hips. Avoid tight-fitting dresses that accentuate your tummy area. Wear a waist-cincher for special occasions to give you more shape. Avoid hipster-style trousers or jeans as these can push the flesh up to create a 'muffin' top of fat and work against your efforts to slim down your waist and abdomen.

Hourglass Shape

Best points
- **Generous bust:** With a heavier bust, a well-fitting bra is essential as it can make you look magnificent. Select a bra with thicker straps to avoid them cutting into your shoulders. Visit a specialist store such as Rigby and Peller (www.rigbyandpeller.co.uk). For tops, wrap-over styles can look great and they will show off your slim waist too. Fitted dresses styled with a small waist are perfect for you. For evening wear, go for something close-fitting and add a belt to a plain dress to show off your curves.
- **Slim waist:** Wear styles that accentuate your lovely waistline. Short, cropped jackets and knits can look good on you.
- **Good legs:** You have fabulous legs, so show them off in most styles of skirt – long or short. Trousers and jeans should be easy for you to wear too. Go for bootleg or straight jeans rather than skinny-leg as you will have wider thighs than an apple shape, but because you have less fat on your thighs compared to a pear shape, you'll be able to wear shorter shorts.
- **Slim ankles:** You are likely to have great ankles, so show them off. Wear high heels when possible and avoid straight-across ankle straps.

Worst points
- **Over-large bust:** With a good bra, even the largest breasts can be controlled into a good shape. Depending on your size, select tops in a style that shows off your bust without it appearing overexposed. Avoid deep-plunge necklines. To make your bust appear smaller, wear dark and plain colours above the waist. Avoid frills and, if you wear anything buttoned across the chest, make sure it's loose enough and doesn't look as if it's about to pop open. Cropped jackets can look great on hourglass shapes as they minimise the bust area.
- **Heavy hips:** Sometimes an hourglass figure can have heavy hips. Careful dressing with smooth lines (no gathers or pleats) can slim them down very effectively. Dark, plain colours work best for this.

GOLDEN RULES FOR DRESSING YOUNGER

- Pastel shades are more flattering to mature skin.
- Have hems and sleeves shortened if necessary. Too-long skirts or cuffs are very ageing.
- Never go out barelegged. Wear fine denier tights to make your legs look naturally suntanned.
- Avoid ankle straps on shoes – they make legs look fatter and shorter.
- High heels make us look slimmer and taller, but make sure you wear a height that's safe for you.
- Wear red if you want to be noticed.
- Wear blue if you want to be remembered.
- Wear shoes the same colour or darker than your outfit.
- Invest in a professional colour consultation to find the best colours for you.
- Avoid mixing textures of fabrics, e.g. wool with linen.
- Recognise your best points and your not-so-good ones and dress accordingly.
- When buying clothes, buy what suits you, not what looks good on the model in a magazine.
- If you are being photographed, try to wear a light colour next to your face, e.g. white or cream, as it reflects light and makes you look younger.
- Avoid being photographed in direct sunlight – it's very unflattering.
- When being photographed, position yourself in a three-quarters position to the camera with your front foot in the 'six o'clock' position and your back foot in the 'ten-past-two' position and placed slightly across – see photograph.

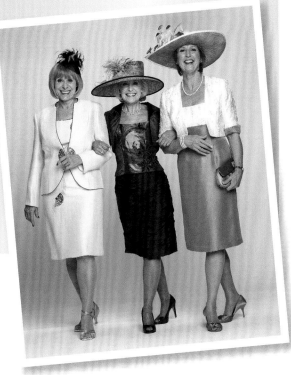

And finally . . .

You know when you are getting old when . . .

- you've been looking for your glasses for half an hour then realise they're on your head
- you can't find your car in the car park
- your husband says, 'Let's go upstairs for sex' and you say, 'I can't do both'
- an 'all-nighter' means that you didn't need to get up in the night to go to the loo!

Your personal calorie allowance (women)

Check against your current weight and age range to find the ideal daily calorie allowance that will give you a healthy rate of weight loss after you've completed the initial four-week diet plan.

Women aged 18–29

Body Weight		(BMR)
Stones	*Kilos*	*Calories*
7	45	1147
7.5	48	1194
8	51	1241
8.5	54	1288
9	57	1335
9.5	60.5	1382
10	64	1430
10.5	67	1477
11	70	1524
11.5	73	1571
12	76	1618
12.5	80	1665
13	83	1712
13.5	86	1760
14	89	1807
14.5	92	1854
15	95.5	1901
15.5	99	1948
16	102	1995
16.5	105	2043
17	108	2090
17.5	111	2137
18	115	2184
18.5	118	2231
19	121	2278
19.5	124	2325
20	127	2373

Women aged 30–59

Body Weight		(BMR)
Stones	*Kilos*	*Calories*
7	45	1108
7.5	48	1144
8	51	1178
8.5	54	1211
9	57	1220
9.5	60.5	1287
10	64	1373
10.5	67	1389
11	70	1414
11.5	73	1440
12	76	1466
12.5	80	1492
13	83	1518
13.5	86	1544
14	89	1570
14.5	92	1595
15	95.5	1621
15.5	99	1647
16	102	1673
16.5	105	1699
17	108	1725
17.5	111	1751
18	115	1776
18.5	118	1802
19	121	1828
19.5	124	1854
20	127	1880

Women aged 60–74

Body Weight		(BMR)
Stones	*Kilos*	*Calories*
7	45	1048
7.5	48	1073
8	51	1099
8.5	54	1125
9	57	1151
9.5	60.5	1176
10	64	1202
10.5	67	1228
11	70	1254
11.5	73	1279
12	76	1305
12.5	80	1331
13	83	1357
13.5	86	1382
14	89	1408
14.5	92	1434
15	95.5	1460
15.5	99	1485
16	102	1511
16.5	105	1537
17	108	1563
17.5	111	1588
18	115	1614
18.5	118	1640
19	121	1666
19.5	124	1691
20	127	1717

Your personal calorie allowance (men)

Check against your current weight and age range to find the ideal daily calorie allowance that will give you a healthy rate of weight loss after you've completed the initial four-week diet plan.

Men aged 18–29

Body Weight		(BMR)
Stones	Kilos	Calories
7	45	1363
7.5	48	1411
8	51	1459
8.5	54	1507
9	57	1555
9.5	60.5	1602
10	64	1650
10.5	67	1698
11	70	1746
11.5	73	1794
12	76	1842
12.5	80	1890
13	83	1938
13.5	86	1986
14	89	2034
14.5	92	2082
15	95.5	2129
15.5	99	2177
16	102	2225
16.5	105	2273
17	108	2321
17.5	111	2369
18	115	2417
18.5	118	2465
19	121	2513
19.5	124	2561
20	127	2609

Men aged 30–59

Body Weight		(BMR)
Stones	Kilos	Calories
7	45	1324
7.5	48	1347
8	51	1387
8.5	54	1425
9	57	1480
9.5	60.5	1527
10	64	1590
10.5	67	1640
11	70	1676
11.5	73	1713
12	76	1749
12.5	80	1786
13	83	1822
13.5	86	1859
14	89	1895
14.5	92	1932
15	95.5	1968
15.5	99	2005
16	102	2041
16.5	105	2078
17	108	2114
17.5	111	2151
18	115	2187
18.5	118	2224
19	121	2260
19.5	124	2297
20	127	2333

Men aged 60–74

Body Weight		(BMR)
Stones	Kilos	Calories
7	45	1232
7.5	48	1270
8	51	1307
8.5	54	1345
9	57	1383
9.5	60.5	1421
10	64	1459
10.5	67	1497
11	70	1535
11.5	73	1573
12	76	1611
12.5	80	1649
13	83	1687
13.5	86	1725
14	89	1763
14.5	92	1801
15	95.5	1839
15.5	99	1877
16	102	1915
16.5	105	1953
17	108	1991
17.5	111	2028
18	115	2066
18.5	118	2104
19	121	2142
19.5	124	2180
20	127	2218

Further information

Rosemary Conley Diet and Fitness Clubs
Find your nearest class at **www.rosemaryconley.com** or call **01509 620620**
Watch our 'at class' video at **www.rosemaryconley.tv/class**

Rosemary Conley's Solo Slim® foods
Order Rosemary Conley's Stay Young Solo Slim® Healthy Food Box on
www.rosemaryconley.com or phone our credit card hotline on **0870 0507727**

Rosemary Conley fitness DVDs and other products
For Rosemary Conley's fitness DVDs, fitness gadgets, Magic Measure®, Toning Band and
Moisturising Firming Cream log on to **www.rosemaryconley.com**

Facial-Flex®
To order log on to **www.rosemaryconley.com**

Rosemary Conley *Diet & Fitness* magazine
To subscribe to the magazine visit **www.rosemaryconley.com** or phone the order hotline on
01509 620444

Online slimming club
To join our online slimming club visit **www.rosemaryconleyonline.com**

Web TV channel
Log on to our web TV channel for free on **www.rosemaryconley.tv**

The Rosemary Conley
ultimate Brush Collection

Professional makeup brushes at sensible prices

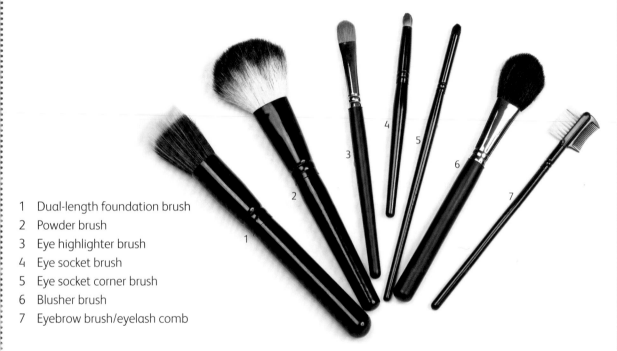

1 Dual-length foundation brush
2 Powder brush
3 Eye highlighter brush
4 Eye socket brush
5 Eye socket corner brush
6 Blusher brush
7 Eyebrow brush/eyelash comb

- Personally tried, tested and selected by Rosemary
- Superb quality
- Easy to use
- Easy to clean
- 90% natural hair*
- Can be purchased individually or as a set

* The white hairs on the dual-length foundation brush are synthetic, as are the bristles in the eyebrow brush/eyelash comb

To order, log on to **www.rosemaryconley.com** or call **0870 0507727**